Winning Over Diabetes

Winning Over Diabetes

Rita Malik
T.K. Malik

Ane Books India

New Delhi ♦ Chennai ♦ Kolkata ♦ Bangalore ♦ Lucknow

Ane Books India

Head Office 4821 Parwana Bhawan, 1st Floor, 24 Ansari Road, Darya Ganj, New Delhi -110002, India,
Tel.: 91(011) 23276843-44, Fax: 91(011) 23276863
e-mail: anebooks@vsnl.com,
Website: www.anebooks.com

Chennai Avantika Niwas, First Floor, 19 Doraiswamy Road, T. Nagar, Chennai - 600017,
Tel.: 91(044) 28141554, 28141209
e-mail: anebooks_tn@airtelbroadband.net

Kolkata Flat No. 16A, 220 Vivekanada Road, Manikatalla, Kolkata - 700006
Tel.: 91(033) 23547119
e-mail: anekol@vsnl.net

Bangalore No. 124, 10th Cross, 29th Main 1st Phase, J.P. Nagar, Bangalore - 560078
Tel. : 91(080) 26536772

Lucknow C-26, Sector-A, Mahanagar, Lucknow - 226006
Mobile - 93352 29971

ISBN 818952126-8

Price : Rs. 150.00

Printed at Shakti Packers, Delhi

Dedication

This book is dedicated to:

- Those who suffer from diabetes,
- Those who are at the risk of developing this disease,
- Those with impaired glucose tolerance.
- To my grandchildren Riya & Gautam.

I wish to reach out to all those afflicted with diabetes and ring the alarm bell before it is too late!

Acknowledgements

We wish to acknowledge our elder son Niten Malik & family who inspired, motivated and encouraged us for writing the book for diabetic patients and general readers. He also went through the manuscript several times and made useful suggestions. We also wish to acknowledge our younger son Dr. Chetan Malik & family who helped us to collect the relevant literature.

We also wish to acknowledge Mr. Partha Maitra (Editor, Hindustan Times) for editing this book and the artist Mr. Sunil Dutt for his realistic diagrams.

At last, we express our sincere thanks to Mr. Sunil Saxena and all the staff member of Ane Books India for their patient help and excellent cooperation.

Rita Malik
T. K. Malik

Preface

Through the ages, the Sadhus, the Rishis, the Babas (Saints and Hermits) of ancient to modern India, have always been a point of discussion for their simple and unique life styles. They lived in mountains, had their dwellings near streams, rivers and springs, derived their food from nature and spent a large chunk of their time meditating. Yoga was yet another most essential part of their life styles. In short, they lived much longer and healthier.

Such a life style may not be possible in today's world. The increased use of fast food and processed food in daily life and the relative lack of exercise in the prevailing life-styles are the root causes of many human ailments. One such ailment is diabetes or 'Sugar Problem' in a layman's language.

I have many friends and relatives who suffer from diabetes. Yet surprisingly, only a few of them take their disease seriously. Majority of them are casual and even reckless about their predicament and come around only when a serious complication hits them.

A friend of mine with diabetes, in spite of repeated warnings, continued to abuse alcohol and indulge in gourmet meals. He ultimately died of kidney failure at the young age of 40.

Another very rich lady of 40, a close relative of ours is not bothered about her own fasting blood sugar level of 291 mg%, but remains worried about her aging mother of 82 years with vertigo.

The poignant purpose of this book is to make each diabetic patient aware of the serious debilitating complications that may afflict his body and how to avoid such mutilating and agonizing conditions in life. The complicated subject of diabetes has been made easy to understand by comprehensive and simple language.

It explains the type of behavioral attitude, which precipitates diabetes in already predisposed ethnic and genetic setting. Through this book, we wish to help generate a better understanding of this complex disease and how it affects just about every organ in the human body. Knowledge is the most effective tool to empower diabetics. The patients should understand and relate to the changes they are required to make in their day to day living.

The information thus gathered make patients better equipped to tackle the situations that may arise from this condition.

This book also details a philosophy, which helps to regulate the life style of a diabetic person. It is not designed to outline the treatment, which should always be determined by the treating doctor. It is a mere theme designed to help you to help yourself.

The salient features of this book are:

- **The first part of the book gives an introduction to the diabetes and details its historical aspects. It also describes the prevalence of the disease, how the body functions normally, as well as its biochemical aspects.**
- **The second part of the book details the common modes of presentation, the types of diabetes, the causes and the complications of diabetes and what goes wrong when a person develops diabetes.**
- **The third part describes how to avoid the disease in a predisposed individual. It also discusses the management of the disease once it becomes manifest. Also, as in this condition all organs of the body are affected, how best to prevent the serious complications. A small portion is devoted to obesity and newer innovations in the field of diabetes. It gives some home remedies and herbs and the health benefits of these natural food articles. It also describes some tasteful Indian recipes that are good for diabetics.**
- **The book contains informatory tables and self explanatory illustrations. These illustrations visually enhance concepts and understanding of the subject.**

Contents

Dedication *v*
Acknowledgements *vi*
Preface *vii*

PART - I

Historical aspects, Incidence & Human Physiology

1. Diabetes is no Disaster **3-5**

- Individual Reactions Towards Diabetes 3
- Accept being Diabetic 3
- Management of Diabetes 4

2. Diabetes Down the Ages **6-8**

This chapter pays homage to the great scientists who made remarkable discoveries and revealed the evolution of the disease from diagnosis to management, over the ages.

- Ancient History of Diabetes 6
- Diabetes in Ayurveda 7
- Discovery of Insulin 8

3. Incidence: Stark Statistics **9-12**

Statistics have shown that cigarette smoking is linked to lung cancer. Statistics of disease help elucidate the causative factors of disease. The incidence of diabetes with respect to ethnic, racial and geographical variations is mentioned herein with their implications.

- Worldwide Incidence of Diabetes 9
- Geographic Incidence 10
- Racial Incidence 10
- Diabetes and Obesity 11
- Necessity of Timely Diagnosis 11

4. Biochemistry **13-26**

Physics and chemistry are basic sciences that form the back - bone of modern technology and has enabled man to land on moon. A little knowledge of biochemistry goes a long way in comprehending the complexities of diabetes.

- Composition of Cells 14
- Hydrocarbons 15
- Bonds Between Atoms 18
- Carbohydrates 19
- Glucose 20
- Fructose 20
- Lactose 20
- Maltose 20
- Sucrose 20
- What is the Relevance of Simple and Complex Carbohydrates with Diabetes? 21
- Glycemic Index (GI) 21
- Proteins 22
- Fats or Lipids 23
- Fatty Acids 23
- Triglycerides 24
- Cholesterol 24
- Digestion, Absorption and Storage of Fats 25

5. Human Physiology: Normal Body Functions **27-31**

It is crucial to imbibe the normal so as to understand the abnormal. This chapter is devoted to the normal functioning of the human system. It does not invade the intricate details but merely skirmishes the surface.

- Digestion of Food we Eat 28
- Absorption of Food 29
- Maintenance of Internal Milieu 31

6. Insulin and its Mode of Action **32-36**

Insulin plays a pivotal role in men's health and well-being. It plays a key role in utilization of sugars by the body. This chapter explains mode of action of insulin, maintenance of blood glucose levels, and regulation of insulin secretion.

- Insulin 32
- Mechanism of Insulin Secretion 33
- Role of Glucagons in Glucose Level Maintenance 34

PART - II

Definition, Etiology & Complications

7. Symptoms of Diabetes **39-41**

The awareness of diabetes is exceedingly low as majority of people are not familiar with the presenting features of the disease. This chapter describes the various modes of presentation of diabetes.

- Symptoms of Diabetes 39
- Type 1diabetes 40
- Type 2diabetes 40
- Impaired Glucose Tolerance 40
- NIDDM and IGT 41
- Lipid Profile 41

8. Definitions and Classification of Diabetes **42-52**

What is diabetes mellitus and what are its different variants? What is the role of heredity in various types of diabetes? What is insulin resistance? What does it imply and is there anything we can do about it? All this is touched upon in the following pages.

- Type 1 DM, IDDM (Insulin Dependent Diabetes Mellitus) 43
- Immune Dysfunction in Type 1diabetes 44
- Genetic Control of Type 1diabetes 45
- Type 2 DM or NIDDM (Non-Insulin Dependent Diabetes Mellitus) 46
- Insulin Resistance 47
- Insulin Resistance in Type 2 DM 47
- Obesity-insulin Resistance Type 2diabetes 48
- PC-1 Protein in Type 2diabetes 48
- Type 1diabetes is More Severe than Type 2 49
- Genetic Research on Diabetes Mellitus 49
- GDM (Gestational Diabetes Mellitus) 50
- Other forms of Diabetes (Secondary Diabetes) 51

9. Diagnosis of Diabetes **53-58**

How to know you have diabetes and how to be absolutely sure that it is not something else? This chapter pertains to who diagnostic criteria, and how to monitor the blood sugar levels?

- Laboratory Tests for Diagnosis of Diabetes 53
- Blood Glucose Test 53
- Glycosylated Haemoglobin (HBA1C) Measurement 54
- Fructosamine Assay 54
- Self-Monitoring of Blood Glucose Level 55
- Glucometer 55
- Glucowatch 55
- Precautions while Using Glucose Meters 57
- Urine Test for Glucose 57
- Hyperglycemia due to other Causes 58

10. Diabetes and Pregnancy and Diabetes and Alcohol 59-63

What precautions to take and what rules to follow when diabetes is associated with pregnancy.
The perverse fascination for alcoholic drinks and relentless decline in simple living has driven man away from nature and made him prey to many ailments. Excessive alcohol wrecks the human body, more so in a diabetic.

- Diabetes in Pregnant Women 59
- Precautions before Conception 60
- Precautions for Diabetic Pregnant Woman 60
- Large Babies 62
- Diabetes and Alcohol 62

11. Pathogenesis of Diabetes 64-72

This chapter briefly describes the role of cardio-vascular system (heart and blood vessels) in preserving the milieu interior (internal environment i.e. the fluid that surrounds and bathes individual cells of body) and then goes on to elaborate the alterations that take place inside the body when a person develops diabetes. It further discusses the consequences of these changes and their role in the development of complications.

- Circulatory System 64
- The Heart 66
- Hypercholesteramia 67
- Atherosclerosis 69
- Arteriosclerosis 69
- Various Physiological Malfunctioning in Diabetes 70
- Somogyi Effect 71

12. Complications of Diabetes **73-94**

The morbidity and mortality of complications of diabetes is so profound that no message is strong enough to beat the menace. The more you know about them the less it is.

- Lipid Disorders 74
- Coronary Heart Disease and Hypertension 74
- Antihypertensive Drugs 74
- Lower Extremity Arterial Disease (LEAD) 76
- Insulin Resistance Syndrome 77
- Diabetic Eye Disease 78
- Diabetic Retinopathy 78
- Cataract 80
- Glaucoma 80
- Kidney Disease 80
- Kidney Function Tests 82
- Structure of Kidney 82
- Non-Healing Wounds 84
- Gangrene 84
- Diabetic Neuropathy 85
- Sensory Disturbances 85
- Motor Disturbances 87
- Autonomic Disturbances 87
- Sexual Dysfunction 88
- Impaired Immunity 90
- Skin Diseases 90
- Dental Complications 90
- Joint Problems 91
- Lactic Acidosis 91
- Hypoglycemia 92
- Diabetic Ketoacidosis 92
- Hyperglycemic, Hyperosmolar, Non Ketotic Syndrome 93

PART - III

Prevention, Management & Newer Innovations

13. Prevention of Diabetes **97-102**

Disease drains energy. The secret to health lies in prevention of disease. Allow not the milk to spill and cry over it. Effort is made herein to discuss the necessary measures.

- Onset of Diabetes 97
- Can we Prevent Diabetes? 98
- Obesity: A Prime Cause of Disease 100
- Greater Risk Category 101
- Precautions for Risk Category 102

14. Let not our Children have Diabetes 103-106

- Type 1diabetes in Children 103
- Type 2diabetes in Children 103
- Obesity and Diabetes 104
- Responsibility of Parents 104
- Precautions During Childhood 105
- Some Considerable Facts 106

15. Management of Diabetes 107-139

A great scientist announced that gene proposes and environment disposes. In other words environment exposes what we inherit. How much of the environment can be handled depends, to quite an extent, on our own activities.

- Diabetes is Mainly a Self-managed Condition 108
- Regime and Treatment of Individual Demands 108
- Hypoglycemia 108
- Care of Feet 109
- Precautionary Measures 110
- Diet Management 110
- Body Weight 111
- Calorie Requirement 113
- Dietary Fiber 114
- Water 114
- Microwater 115
- Proteins 116
- Plant Proteins 116
- Animal Proteins 117
- Carbohydrate Intake and Vigil 117
- Artificial Sweeteners 117
- Natural Sweeteners 118
- Fatty Alarm 119
- Saturated Fatty Acids 119

- Unsaturated Fatty Acids 119
- Vitamins 120
- Need for Vitamins 120
- Vitamin A 121
- Vitamin B 121
- Anti Oxidants : The Protective Shield 124
- Some Antioxidants 124
- Diet for Diabetics 127
- Exercise 129
- Yoga or Yogic Exercises 131
- Breathing Exercises 131
- Corpse Position 132
- Abdominal Breathing 132
- Alternate Nostril Breathing 133
- Kapalabhati 133
- Double Leg Lift 134
- Forward Bend 134
- Side Bend 135
- Spine Twist 135
- Anaerobic Exercise 136
- Duration of Exercise 137
- Advantages of Exercise 137
- Planning Exercise 138

16. Obesity **140-145**

How to tackl2diabetes It is a million dollar question. The causes and management of obesity is discussed in the following pages.

- Management of Obesity 140
- Biology of Hunger 141
- Chemical Messengers to Control Hunger 141
- Mental Attitude 143
- Lose Weight Live Healthy 144

17. Management of Stress **146-149**

Stress is an elusive phenomenon. At times circumstances are such2diabetesss becomes inevitable. The following paragraphs discuss the generation of stress and how to negate it.

- Excessive Desires-the Root Cause of Stress 146
- How Does One Deal with Stress? 147
- Influence of Prayer on Stress 148
- Benefits of Prayer 148
- Effect of Meditation on Stress 148
- Other Methods to Relieve Stress 149

18. Medication **150-156**

2diabetestion should be the last resort. But if the doctor prescribes it do not avoid it.

- Oral Pills 150
- Sulphonylureas 151
- Biguanides 152
- Alpha-Glucosidase Inhibitors 152
- Thiazolidinediones 152
- Actos 153
- Repaglinide 153
- D-phenylalanine Derivatives 154
- Insulin 154
- Site of Insulin Injection 155

19. Home Remedies **157-161**

. Herbs and certain food ingredients that are helpful in diabetes are mentioned herein.

- Ginger 157
- Indian Gooseberry 157
- Jamun 158
- Bitter Gourd or Plant Insulin 158
- Fenugreek 158
- Black Gram 158
- Guar 158
- Curry Leaves 159
- Barley 159
- Fruits 159
- Groundnut 159
- Holy Basil 159
- Ancient Drugs used in Diabetes 160
- Gugolipid 160
- Gymnema Sylvestre 161

20. Recent Advances in Diabetes **162-167**

It is always rewarding to keep informed. Some of the recent research and discoveries are mentioned below.

- Transplant Surgery 162
- Trials on Transplant Surgery 162
- Obstructions in Transplant Surgery 163
- Genetic Engineering Research in Transplant Surgery 163
- Insulin Therapy 164
- Leptin Injection 164
- Regranex 165
- AGEs 166
- C-peptide 166
- Atorvastatin 166
- New Drugs on Clinical Trial 167

21. Recipes for Diabetics **168-185**

- Lassi 169
- Nimbu Adrak Pani 169
- Adrak Elaichi Tea 170
- Raita 170
- Sooji Uppma 171
- Palak Paneer 172
- Ginger Garlic Halibut 173
- Spinach Salmon 173
- Ginger Lime Salmon 174
- Tandoori Chicken 174
- Roasted Chicken 175
- Bitter Gourd 176
- Onion Okra 177
- Urad Dal 178
- Red Kidney Beans 179
- Kaboli Chana 180
- Kala Chana 181
- Sambar 182
- Punjabi Kadhi 183
- Sarson Ka Saag 184
- Sandesh 185

References *186-189*

PART - I

Historical aspects, Incidence & Human Physiology

Chapter 1

DIABETES IS NO DISASTER

"I know nothing except the fact of my ignorance"

Socrates

Can we turn back the clock in our lives to a time, when disease stalks in the silent garb of diabetes? It is silent because it does not rain havoc but eats away like rust. A disease that depletes the body and devastates every vital organ, being a bitter life partner. Yet, diabetes is not a fate accompli. Yes, you can turn back the clock and start on the path to a healthy, long life. The 'mantra'* is to make sensible workable changes in life style.

Individual Reaction Towards Diabetes

When a person is first diagnosed as diabetic, the initial feeling is one of alarm or even shock and depression. After the initial reaction, the sinking feeling gives way to reconciliation and acceptance. While some patient gear up to face the challenge, others fail to perceive the gravity of the situation and remain indifferent and careless. Perhaps, they lack the knowledge of the consequences of this disorder. Some are under the misconception that their disease is mild and they tend to take liberties. Diabetes is no disaster. Yet it should be treated seriously.

Accept Being Diabetic

There is **no need for denial and there is no need for despair.** What matters most at this stage is the person's attitude, determination and motivation to face the disease and make the necessary life style changes? There is no reason to feel depressed or hindered or handicapped. Among the many famous people, who had diabetes include *Ernest Hemmingway, H.G.Wells, Elizabeth Taylor* and *Elvis Presley*. They have done wonders in their lifetime, so why can't you and I? Actually, the discovery of diabetes should make the patient lead a more disciplined life, leading to a better quality of life. He must set to realign his life style and activities. By doing so, he delays the process of ageing and certainly delays the onset of complications.

At this point, he needs the **support of his family** and **friends,** as diabetes is a life long disorder with many complications. The patient must understand all facets of the disease so that they are able to take the necessary measures to lead a healthy life and remain free of the complications, which is a strong motivating factor.

The human mind is a marvelous instrument. It can undertake any endeavor and can achieve any objective it sets its mind to. The mind can look after the body. But, it needs to be enlightened with knowledge to carry out its functions. The functions of the body are intricately designed, delicately interwoven, and finely tuned. A very small defect can put the entire machinery out of gear and in chaos. The exploration and insight in this discipline of medicine has steadily contributed to a growing knowledge base. It guides and inspires the scientists to lead to concrete improvement in the management, survival and quality of life of the diabetics. In this age of science, explorative insight and research initiatives has brought in an era of hope. However, the knowledge of diabetes is imperative for good **self-management** by the patient, under the guidance of a medical professional.

Management of Diabetes

Diabetes is a **life long disorder,** which is markedly affected by day-to-day variations in diet, exercise, infection and stress. These factors have to be addressed on daily basis while managing diabetes and the patient is the person best equipped to deal with the situation. Hence, a thorough knowledge of the disease and how it alters normal body functions and the awareness of its acute and chronic complications is necessary. It enables the diabetic patient to take better care of him or herself. Awareness of diabetes, its complications and better health care has proved to improve the long-term outlook of this disease.

The management of diabetes is intimately linked to food. Therefore, knowledge about food and nutrition and the scientific base of biochemistry, physiology, and pathogenesis** go a long way towards the understanding and dealing with this disorder. The following chapters explore all aspects of disease and its management. All the chapters combined, weave into a comprehensive text and over the pages a more complete picture of the diabetic state and its management emerges.

---

* Mantra means key message or a code or secret.

** Pathos refers to abnormal state and genesis signifies generation, hence, pathogenesis means the development of abnormal state.

Chapter 2

DIABETES DOWN THE AGES

"Those who fail to read history are destined to suffer from the repetition of mistakes."

This chapter pays homage to the great scientists who made remarkable discoveries in this field. They revealed the evolution of the disease from diagnosis to management, over the ages. Ancient Indian, Romans, Chinese and Greeks recognized diabetes. In the *Ayurvedic* literature, reference has been made to the disease, as long back as 1000 B.C. *Sushrata*, an ancient Indian and eminent surgeon was the first to identify diabetes and linked it to something wrong in the blood. In the late 19th century, two German scientists made landmark discoveries. Later, *Fredrick Banting* and *Charles Best* discovered insulin. The continuing research has led to the formation of synthetic human insulin. Gene mapping, genetic engineering and pancreatic transplantation are frontiers of research in the modern era.

Ancient History of Diabetes

Diabetes mellitus has worldwide distribution, highly prevalent in both developing and developed countries. Diabetes is an ancient predicament, which has afflicted many, over the ages cutting across geographic and racial barriers. It was recognized more than 2000 years ago. The Romans found that patients suffering from this condition, to pass sweet tasting urine. The Latin word for sweet being **mellitus.** The Greeks found such patients to pass urine as rapidly as they drank water, as if it was getting siphoned out. The Greek word for siphon being **diabetes**. Hence, this disease assumed a unique nomenclature, straddling two civilizations and was called **diabetes mellitus.** Some important earlier discoveries are listed below.

- In 1500 BC, *Papyrus Ebrs* an Eygptian used remedies for the patients passing too much urine.
- Arabian writers translated information about diabetes from ancient Indian text.
- Greek physicians (275-230 BC) diagnosed diabetes and associated with the weakness of kidneys, loss of water and dehydration and used pot herbs such as lettuce, rockfish and juice of knotgrass as remedies.
- In 1622-1675 AD, *Sushrata's* work was recognized where he described diabetes as disease of blood due to hormonal changes.
- In 1798 AD, *John Rolls* showed that in diabetes, there is excess sugar in blood.
- *L. Trube* (1816-1876), showed link between carbohydrate intake and presence of sugar in urine.
- In late 19th century, with Western science making giant leaps in research and exploration, a vital breakthrough was achieved.

Diabetes in Ayurveda

In the **Ayurvedic** literature, reference has been made to a disease resembling diabetes as far back as 1000 BC referred as *Prameha*. It details a condition where urine is passed excessively both in quantity and frequency. In Sanskrit, the prefix ***Pra*** means excessive in both frequency and quantity and ***Meha*** means watering. In the Sanskrit text, *prameha* is further classified and one of the types is referred to as ***Madhumeha***. The prefix ***madhu*** means sweet, hence the word *madhumeha* refers to a disease more closely resembling diabetes mellitus. The etiology, pathogenesis and treatment of diabetes mellitus mentioned in the Ayurvedic text are astonishingly similar to the modern concepts of diabetes. The description of two types of *madhumeha*, the **lean diabetic** and the **obese diabetic** in Vedic classification is strikingly similar to the **modern type 1** and **type** 2diabetes. Similarly, there is reference to the congenital variant (*sahaja prameha*—due to defective seed) and *apathyanimitthaja prameha i.e.* due to overeating and wrong eating habits. Two stalwarts of ancient Indian medicine, *Charaka* and *Sushrata* have written extensively on madhumeha. *Charaka* was a very able and renowned physician and *Sushrata* was an equally competent surgeon. He was the first to diagnose diabetes. Both have many treaties to their credit. These were called ***samhitas*** in Sanskrit. The word *madhumeha* has also been used, in their texts with reference to diabetes. *Madhumeha* is more appropriate term for diabetes. *Sushrata* has devoted one complete chapter to the treatment of *madhumeha*, in his book. He considered it a more complicated form of *prameha*. At that time, when modern investigations were not known, diabetes insipidus, an endocrinal disorder, in which also excessive urine is passed, was considered a distinct type of *prameha*.

Discovery of Insulin

In 1889, two German scientists discovered that a dog whose pancreas had been removed accidentally passed sugar in urine. Later, *Joseph von Mering* and *Oskar Minkowski* proved that pancreatic hormonal secretion controlled the use of sugar by the body. This hormone secreted by the pancreas is called **insulin**. *Dr. Frederick Banting* and *Charles Best* discovered insulin in 1921. In 1923, *John J.R. Macleod* and *Frederick Banting* won the Nobel Price in medicine for their work. Thirty years later, *Frederick Sanger* defined the amino acid sequence of bovine insulin and got the Nobel prize in chemistry.

The pioneering research has led to the formation of synthetic human insulin. **Gene mapping***, **Genetic engineering**** and pancreatic transplantation are the frontiers of research in modern era.

---

* Gene mapping is location of genes on the chromosomes.

** Genetic engineering is gene manipulation by highly technical procedures.

Chapter 3

Incidence: Stark Statistics

"The numbers are increasing and touching epidemic proportions."

Statistics of disease help to elucidate the causative factors of disease. By virtue of statistics, it has been ascertained that cigarette smoking is linked to lung cancer. This chapter explains the incidence of diabetes with respect to ethnic, racial and geographical variations with their implications. The effect of rich fatty food and sedentary life style on the development of diabetes is also discussed.

Statistics is not just mere numbers. It is a powerful tool. It reveals the past, gives insight into the evolution of the disease and predicts the future. This chapter describes prevalence of the disease based on geographic variance, ethnic and racial groups and socioeconomic status. The data, thus obtained, throws light on the etiology and evolution of the disease. It also gives the prevalence rate of the complications affecting this condition.

Worldwide Incidence of Diabetes

Millions of people all over the world suffer from diabetes. It is estimated that about 200 million persons around the world have diabetes. As per projected estimates, the global prevalence is likely to touch 360 million marks by the year 2030. In America, there are about 21 million people with diabetes and the number is rapidly increasing. Of the estimated 21 million, around 2 million are type 1diabetes mellitus (DM) and the remaining are mostly type 2. For all the ages, 90% of people with diabetes have type 2, but at age greater than 45 years, virtually all people with diabetes have type 2. Type 1 is one of the most common chronic diseases in children in USA and its incidence is increasing around the world.

For all ages, the incidence of diagnosed diabetes is equal or slightly higher in women.

Between 1990 and 2001, US government survey showed diabetes cases almost doubling among people aged 30 to 50. These numbers are increasing by half in the age group of 18 to 29.

Geographic Incidence

There is a remarkable variation in the geographic incidence of diabetes. The incidence of type 1DM is 0.7 per 100,000 in Shanghai, China, while it is 26 times greater in *Whites* in Allegheny County, PA, (18.2 per 100,000) and more than 50 times greater in Finland (35.3 per 100,000).

India may be the diabetes capital of world. India has been projected by the WHO as the country with the fastest growing number of diabetics. In the year 2000, a survey carried out by the ICMR (Indian Council of Medical Research) showed that India has approximately 32 million diabetic patients in a population of over 1 billion. Worse still, the figure is estimated to shoot up to *57 million by 2025*. Research conducted in Madras on 26,000 people, who were more than 20 years old, showed that at least 12% of them had diabetes. About half of the affected people suffered from hypertension but did not even know that they had the disease. The research director said, "Awareness levels are appalling low."

Racial Incidence

There are racial and ethnic variations also. It is possible that ethnic and familial clustering is a result of both, shared genes, and shared behavior and environmental risk factors.

Type 1 is more common in *Whites* and *Hispanics* as compared to the African, Americans and Mexican Americans. However, Type 2 has higher prevalence in African Americans, Mexican Americans and Native Americans compared to non-Hispanic whites.

Among the different people, the incidence is higher in African-Americans, Hispanics, Asians and Native Americans. It is estimated that about 25% of cases of diabetes are present in minorities in the USA.

Diabetes and Obesity

As affluence is increasing in poor countries like India and China, so also is the incidence of diabetes, in these countries. Diabetes is linked to obesity, which can be linked to sedentary lifestyle and fast food fad, which is the fallout of growing affluence. As wealth flows in a family, the food becomes rich and fatty. The sedentary habits creep in, so individuals become obese and develop the tendency of getting diabetes.

Grim or smiling, the obese Sumo wrestlers make good television show and even trigger packed houses. The grim reality is that more than 40% of these Japanese wrestlers are diabetics, while the incidence of diabetes is low in Japan. The prevalence of diabetes in Japan is approximately 3%. The bottom line is that, **obesity is the root cause of diabetes** in the world. Also, the Japanese, who have migrated to America and adopted the eating habits of the community therein have also acquired their rate of incidence.

Necessity of Timely Diagnosis

Many cases remain undiagnosed and unnoticed. It is estimated that the number of undiagnosed cases equals the diagnosed cases of diabetes. The number of cases with impaired glucose tolerance (IGT) is even more than the undiagnosed cases of diabetes. The prevalence of people with IGT follows similar trends as seen for NIDDM (non-insulin dependent diabetes mellitus) and similar variation exists in racial and ethnic groups. In the age group of 20-44 years, the prevalence ranges from 5.5% in non-Hispanic whites to 10.8% in African Americans.

A number of new patients are adding to the list everyday. It is believed that about 800,000 new cases of diabetes add to the list every year. In America, 54,000 die from diabetes related causes. Many are diagnosed at the time of development of some complication or the other, such as blindness.

Diabetes is a major risk factor for heart disease, stroke and amputation. It shortens the lifespan, on an average, up to 15 years and it is the 6th leading cause of death.

The risk of heart disease is two to four times more common in patients with diabetes, as also the risk of stroke. It is the leading cause of blindness and accounts for 40% of end stage renal disease.

David Loshak in his review, in the American Journal of Preventive Medicine, has indicated that nearly three-quarters of adult diabetics in the United States have hypertension and regardless of age, sex and ethnic origin, each patient benefits from efforts to prevent and control it. According to the recent estimates, the prevalence of diabetes in the USA is predicted to be **8.9 percent** of the population by the year 2025.

Chapter 4

BIOCHEMISTRY

'It is good to know about elements for it is elementary in the understanding of anything worth its salt."

Physics and chemistry form the back-bone of modern technology. A little knowledge of biochemistry goes a long way in comprehending the complexities of diabetes. We eat, drink, sleep and work and consider it as a matter of fact. But we are not aware how the millions of cells that constitute our body make it happen. The individual cells live and function to make us live, work and survive. The foods that we eat namely fats, proteins and carbohydrates are complex compounds. In this chapter, the structure of simple molecules is explained in a manner that leads to the understanding of complex molecules and as well as those of lipoproteins that play a significant role in the genesis of many diseases in the body.

The human body is composed of millions of small microscopic (as you need a microscope to see them) basic units called **cells**. These cells derive energy from a type of sugar called **glucose**. We know how kids get a boost of energy when they eat chocolates. Similarly, the cells in the body get energy by using **glucose**. The process of utilizing glucose is called metabolism. It is this **metabolism**, which gets affected in diabetes.

The human body is made of cells and the cells are made of elements found in nature. Two or more elements combine to form substances called **compounds**. These compounds are classified into two broad categories- inorganic compounds and organic compounds. The inorganic compounds include different types of salts such as sodium chloride (common salt) and sodium hydroxide, an alkali. Organic compounds are made of two common elements, carbon and hydrogen. Foods such as proteins, fats and carbohydrates are examples of organic compounds.

Composition of Cells

Water, a molecule made of hydrogen and oxygen is an integral and important constituent of each and every cell of the body. It is also the basic constituent of blood and other fluids in the body. It constitutes more than 70% of the total body mass. Calcium and phosphates, along with other inorganic elements form an integral part of cells of bones and teeth of the body. Human blood, like all other organs in the body, is also made of cells. Among them are red blood cells, which help to carry oxygen from the lungs to all parts of the body. Iron, another element, is a major inorganic component of the hemoglobin present in red blood cells of the body. Similarly, copper, zinc, selenium, molybdenum and other elements are important and found in varying quantities in cells throughout the body. Some form integral constituents of the tissues of the body and some act as catalysts for the myriads of metabolic reactions that take place in the cells of the body. Remember reading the label on the back of a multi-vitamin bottle. You will see some of these inorganic compounds and elements the body needs.

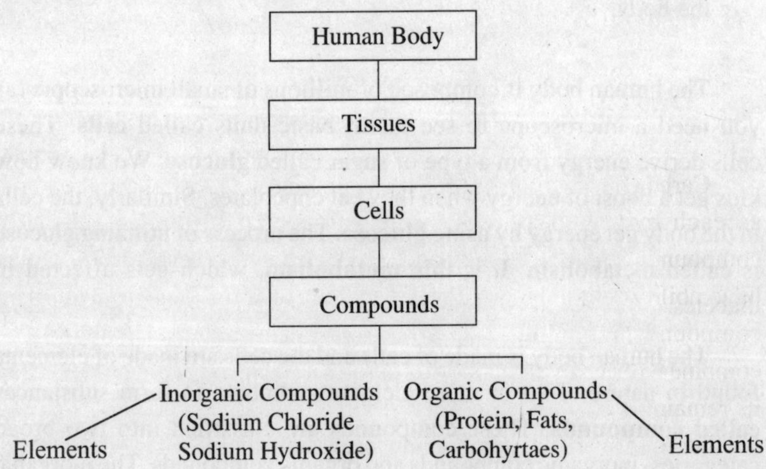

Fig. 4.1 Organisation of human body

Hydrocarbons

Proteins, fats and carbohydrates are the three major organic compounds that constitute the human body. Proteins, fats and carbohydrates are hydrocarbons. These organic compounds are derivatives of hydrocarbons. Hydrocarbons are compounds made up of elements, **hydrogen** and **carbon**. These elements are made of small particles called **atoms**. Each atom has its own combining capacity called its **valence**. Hydrogen has a single valence whereas carbon has four. Another way of describing this is that carbon has 4 hooks or hands and hydrogen has only one. Thus, carbon has the ability to hold 4 hydrogen atoms by the virtue of its 4 hooks. Thus, one carbon atom combines with four hydrogen atoms to form a stable compound. The carbon atoms can also link with one another. They may get linked to one another to either form simple and/or complex straight chain compounds or join one another to form cyclic chains or ring-shaped molecules.

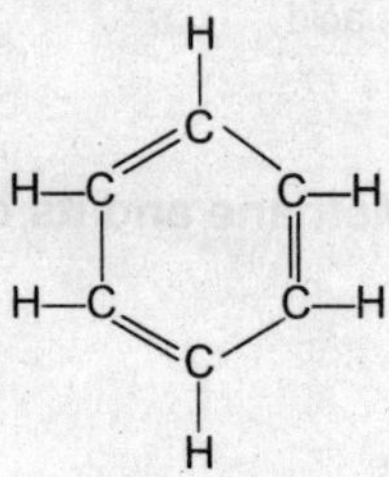

Benzene

Fig. 4.2 Benzene-a ring shaped molecule

Carbon having four valences can combine with four hydrogen atoms as each hydrogen atom has one valence to form straight chain compounds e.g. CH_4 – methane, C_2H_6- ethane. These carbon atoms have ability to combine with one another to form long straight chain compounds, e.g. C–C–C–C. This four-chain carbon compound can combine with ten hydrogen atoms to form a stable molecule by saturating its remaining ten valences. The carbon atoms can also combine to one another to form cyclic compounds instead of straight chain compounds such as benzene.

CH_4	Methane	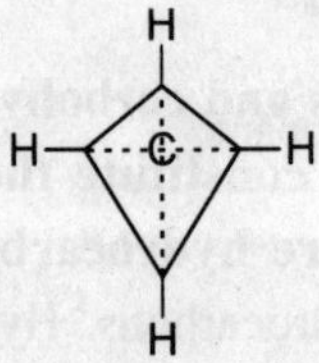 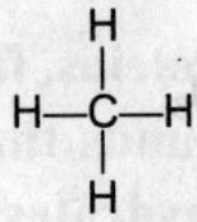
CH_4	Methane	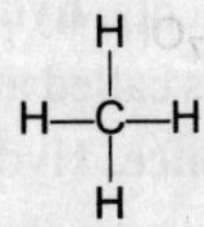
CH_3OH	Methanol or methyl alcohol	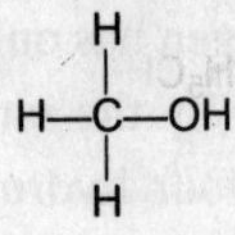
$HCHO$	Formaldehyde	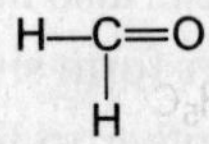
$HCOOH$	Formic acid	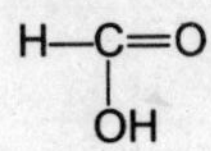

Fig. 4.3 Methane and its derivatives

C_2H_6	Ethane	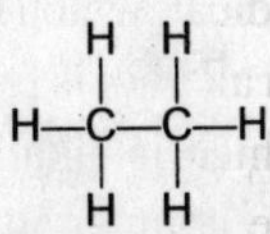
C_2H_5OH	Ethanol or ethyl alcohol	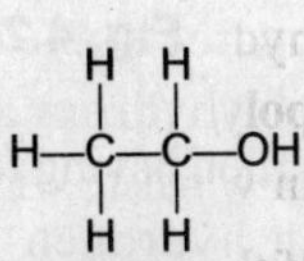
CH_3CHO	Acetaldehyde	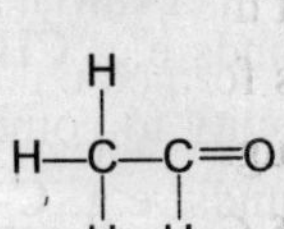
CH_3COOH	Acetic acid	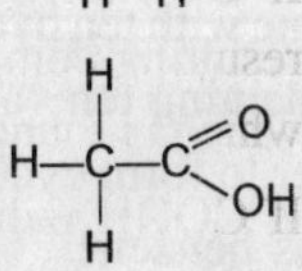

Fig. 4.4 Ethane and its derivatives

C_3H_8 Propane

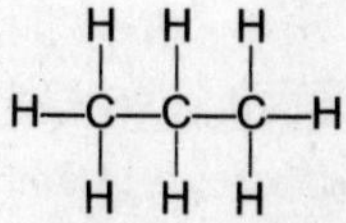

C_3H_7OH Propanol or propyl alcohol

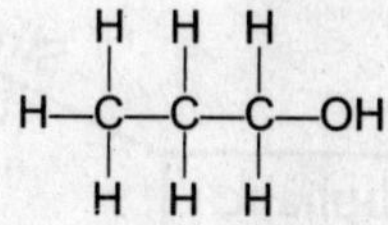

C_2H_5CHO Propyl aldehyde

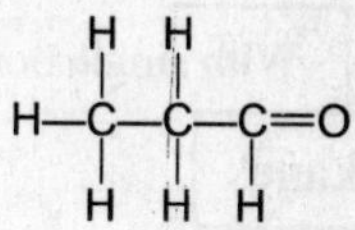

C_2H_5COOH Propanic acid

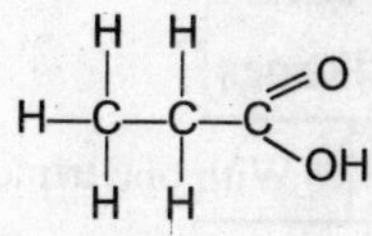

Fig. 4.5 Propane and its derivatives

If one atom of hydrogen in a hydrocarbon is replaced by OH radical, which is called **hydroxyl group** and is also monovalent, an alcohol is formed e.g. OH–CH_3 (methyl alcohol) a compound which is alkali in nature. **Methyl alcohol** is spirit found over the counter in pharmacy and used to clean wounds. When a hydrocarbon has multiple hydroxyl radicals, it is called a **polyhydroxy alcohol**. Ethyl alcohol, an another alcohol is found in whisky, wines and perfumes.

- If the hydrogen atom is replaced by CHO radical, an aldehyde, is formed e.g. CH_3CHO (ethyl aldehyde). These are found in sugar, wheat, rice and other carbohydrates.
- If CO radical (a ketone group), replaces the hydrogen, the resulting compound is ketone. Example of ketone is *acetone*, which is found in nail polish.
- If COOH radical (an acid group), replaces the hydrogen, the resulting compound is a fatty acid. Fatty acid is a type of fat which is found in our diet and in our body.

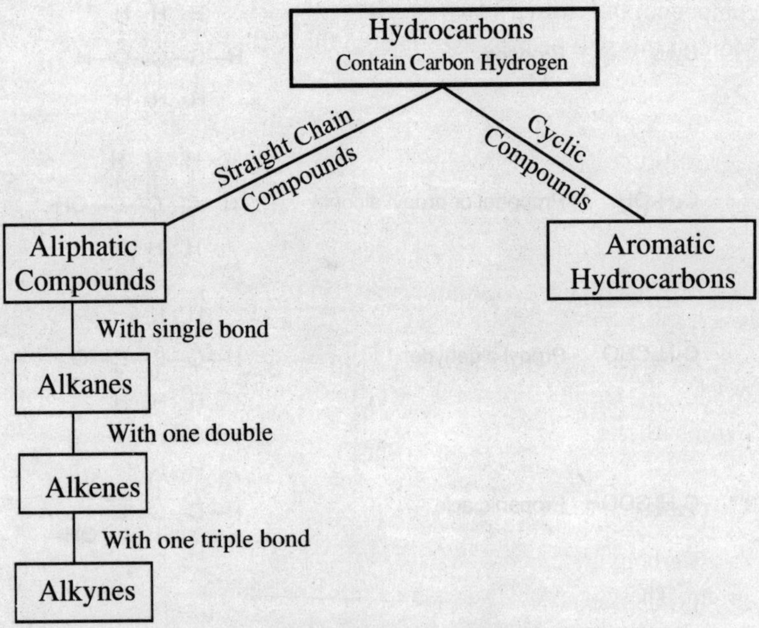

Fig. 4.6 Representation of hydrocarbons

Bonds Between Atoms

As we know two or more elements combine to form compounds. The elements combine with one another through links, which are also called bonds. The bonds are important to form stable compounds.

If the bond between two carbon atoms is a single bond and the remaining valences are satisfied by other radicals or groups the compound is called a **saturated compound**. However, if there are two or more bonds between the carbon atoms, the resulting compound is called an **unsaturated compound**. This is more important and relevant with respect to fats and fatty acids. A fatty acid with single double bond is called a **monounsaturated fatty acid**. The fatty acid with multiple double bonds is called a **polyunsaturated fatty acid**. The consumption of saturated fats as found in butter and ghee, is unhealthy and predisposes to heart attacks, stroke and hypertension. While oils such as olive oil, canola oil and other vegetable oils have higher amounts of unsaturated fatty acids and are healthier.

A compound with 10 carbon atoms is often referred to as 10-C compound, one with 12 carbon atoms as 12-C compound and so on. More of this will be discussed later in the text.

C_2H_3COOH Unsaturated acid

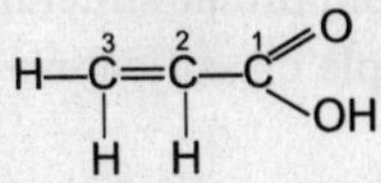

Prop (2 & 3) en 1-oic acid
(propenoic acid)

Fig. 4.7 Propenoic acid, an unsaturated acid

Now let us learn specifically about three major constituents of food i.e., **Carbohydrates, Proteins** and **Fats**, which are all hydrocarbons.

Carbohydrates

Carbohydrates are **polyhydroxy alcohols** with aldehyde or ketone group. These Carbohydrates are simple or complex in nature. Simple carbohydrates are often referred to as sugars, e.g. naturally occurring sugars found in honey, milk, fruits, bread and table sugar. Simple sugars, which are made of single units of 6 carbon compound, are called **monosaccharides**. Examples of monosaccharides are glucose as found in honey and fructose as found in fruits. Glucose found in blood is the primary source of energy for cells. Simple sugars with two 6-carbon units combine to form diasaccharides. Examples of disaccharides are maltose found in malt, lactose found in milk, sucrose in sugarcane or table sugar. Sugar found in human blood is glucose and in the following text, blood glucose is often referred to as blood sugar.

Table 4.1 Types of carbohydrates and their examples.

Types of Carbohydrate	Composition	Examples
Monosaccharides	Simple sugars	Glucose, Galactose, fructose
Disaccharides	Two simple sugars in one molecule	Sucrose (table sugar), maltose, lactose
Polysaccharides	Many monosacch-aride units	Starch, glycogen (animal starch), cellulose

Polysaccharides are complex sugars. Example includes glycogen, which is a polymer of glucose, and is found in liver and muscle cells. Glycogen is the storage form of glucose. Complex carbohydrates also form important structural component of cells such as cell membrane. A simple classification of carbohydrates is given in the table below.

Glucose

It is a naturally occurring sugar present in honey. It causes a fast and high rise in blood glucose levels when ingested. All carbohydrates, when eaten, break down mostly into monosaccharides during digestion in the intestine and before their absorption. Glucose is the main fuel from which the body derives its energy.

It is important to know that nerve cells present in the brain and spinal cord, largely depend on glucose for their energy requirements.

Whenever, the blood glucose level exceeds 180 mg%, the glucose starts getting excreted into the urine, as the renal threshold for glucose is 180 mg%.

Fructose

Fructose is the commonly occurring natural sugar present in fruits and honey. It does not cause high-rise in blood sugar levels, when ingested. It is sweeter than cane sugar. Honey is natural syrup that contains about 35% glucose and about 40% fructose.

Lactose

It is made of one molecule each of glucose and galactose linked together. It is the sugar present in milk. It is less sweet than cane sugar.

Maltose

It is made of two molecules of glucose linked together. It is less sweet than cane sugar.

Sucrose

It is the cane sugar and is made of one molecule each of glucose and fructose. It is present naturally in sugarcane and sugar beet.

What is the Relevance of Simple and Complex Carbohydrates with Diabetes?

The simple carbohydrates such as monosaccharides and disaccharides are easily and quickly digested and get rapidly absorbed from the intestine into the blood, resulting in a quick and high rise in blood sugar levels. This is not good in a diabetic, as the patient is unable to handle a heavy load of glucose at the same speed as a normal person. Moreover, high levels of blood sugar persist for a longer periods of time in diabetics. Hence, it is advisable for a diabetic not to eat those articles of food, which are rich in simple sugars such as cane sugar, mangoes and candy, at least not in high quantities. Complex carbohydrates, in contrast are digested and absorbed over a longer period of time and are therefore better suited in a diabetic patient. The complex sugars are present in whole-wheat grain, grams, oat, barley and lentils. **Glycogen** is a polymer of glucose. Several glucose units join together to form a large molecule of glycogen.

Glycemic Index (GI)

Some years ago, it was realized that different carbohydrates on ingestion, raise blood sugar levels to different degrees, although the calorie value is same. The extent to which the level of blood glucose goes up on eating a particular food item is called its **glycemic index**. The glycemic index uses white bread as the base line, which is given the value of 100. If another food item of the same calorie value on ingestion raises the blood glucose level to half, the level of white bread then the GI [glycemic index] of that substance is 50, which is half that of white bread. **Honey** has a **lower GI** as compared to cane sugar, so if you must eat sugar than eat honey. Certain food items such as whole grain bread, unrefined cereals as oats, pasta, basmati rice, legumes and lentils have low GI in comparison to white bread, cornflakes, cakes, cookies, muffins and icecream. Fruits such as grapes, mangoes and banana have higher GI as compared to apple, plums, guava, papaya and cantaloupes. Diabetic patient should **preferably consume** food items with **lower glycemic index**.

Table 4.2 Glycemic index (GI) of some food items.

Food Items	GI	Food Items	GI
Ice cream	61	Pear	36
Raisins	64	Grapes	43
Cake	67	Oranges	43
Croissant	67	Plum	24
Soft drink	68	Grapefruit	25
Mars bar	68	Peaches	28
Muffin	69	Tomato	38
Potato mashed	70	Yogurt	14
Bagel	72	Milk skim	32
Pop corn	72	Soybeans	18
French fries	73	Split peas	33
Donut	76	Lentils	29
Waffle	76	Tortilla	38
Glucose	102	Honey	73
Maltose	105	White bread	69
Sucrose	65	Rice instant	87
Pineapple	66	Pizza cheese	60
Banana	53	Mixed grain	45
Mango	55	Pasta	45
Apple	36		

Table adapted from the American Journal of Clinical Nutrition 62 (1995): 871-935.

Proteins

Proteins are also organic compounds and constitute an innate portion of the structure and composition of our body. These form the muscles of the body and also integral component of all cells of the body. The building blocks of proteins are amino acids. The amino acids are **radicals**, which contain nitrogen. There are several types of amino acids. Some of these amino acids can be produced in the body from other organic substances, while others cannot be produced. Those that can be synthesized by the body are called **non-essential amino acids**, while those that cannot be synthesized and need to be consumed in the food are called **essential amino acids**. Hormones, enzymes and antibodies are some of the common protein molecules.

- Hormones are substances that control many functions of the body. For example, sex hormones are responsible for all reproductive functions, including production of ova in females and sperms in males. Insulin, a hormone secreted by the pancreas controls metabolism of glucose.
- Enzymes are biological catalysts which speed up a chemical reaction in the body. For example, enzymes are substances present in digestive juices in stomach and intestine that help in the digestion of food.
- Antibodies are substances secreted by cells of the immune system of the body. These fight with germs that may invade the body causing disease.

Thus, proteins are critical for the health, structure and function of the body.

Fats or Lipids

If you put a drop of oil in water it will not mix with it. This is the defining property of fats. Fats are substances which are not soluble in water but soluble in organic solvents such as chloroform, benzene, xylene, etc.

The common fats include fatty acids, triglycerides, (compounds of glycerol, a base and fatty acids) and cholesterol.

Fatty Acids

Fatty Acids are compounds that contain COOH radical. They are present in cooking oil. If you study carefully the label on cooking oil you may read words like linolenic acid or stearic acid. These are different types of fatty acids. The fatty acids have variable length and number of carbon atoms, but quite a few are 16, 18 and even longer chain carbon compounds. Cells also use fatty acids as fuel to obtain energy. Fats are the store houses of energy. When a person starves and his glycogen stores are depleted, he utilizes fats for his energy requirements.

Triglycerides

These are another type of fats found in nature. They are made of **fatty** acids and **glycerol**. Glycerol is what is commonly called glycerine, the sweet substance often used to make ice creams.

Cholesterol

Cholesterol is a heavy and dense molecule. It is a complex compound found widely in nature. It is present in the yellow of eggs. It is an important raw material used by the body in the synthesis of several end products such as steroids and sex hormones.

As fats are not soluble in water, these cannot be transported in their native form in the blood, as blood is a water-based fluid. To enable fats to be carried in the circulation, a protein layer is required to coat them, making them water-soluble. These complexes are called **lipoproteins**. Here, protein is like an envelope holding fats within it. Thus, lipoproteins are tiny packets where the envelope is made of protein and the contents are fats such as cholesterol, triglycerides and fatty acids.

As cholesterol is denser compared to triglycerides, there is more cholesterol in HDL (High Density Lipoproteins) and less in LDL (Low Density Lipoproteins) and VLDL (Very Low Density Lipoproteins) and there is more of triglycerides in chylomicrons as compared to other lipoproteins

Those packets that contain more triglycerides and less cholesterol are lighter and are called low density lipoproteins. Thus, on the basis of their weight and density, lipoproteins are classified into-HDL, LDL, VLDL, and chylomicrons. HDL is a small dense molecule, while LDL is bigger and lighter than HDL and VLDL is still bigger and lighter and chylomicrons are the lightest and the largest.

Table 4.3 Composition of the lipoproteins in human plasma.

Fractions	Source	Density	Proteins%	Total Lipids%
Chylomicrons	Intestine	Less than 0.96	1-2	98-99
VLDL	Liver and intestine	0.96-1.006	7-10	90-93
LDL	Liver and intestine	1.019-1.063	21	79
HDL	Liver and intestine	1.063-1.125	33	67

Digestion, Absorption and Storage of Fats

Fats taken in meals are digested, absorbed in the intestine and then transported in the circulation as chylomicrons and are later carried to the liver. These are rapidly metabolized in the liver and converted to other types of fats such as HDL and LDL, which are then returned to the circulation.

Fats that are stored in fat depots in the body such as subcutaneous tissue, inside the abdomen in the mesentery and omentum, are mostly triglycerides. LDL are considered harmful to the body and HDL are found to be protective in nature, as high levels of LDL in the blood have been found associated with the increased risk of heart attack and stroke and the opposite holds true with the HDL. The reason being that LDL being a bigger and lighter molecule it gets trapped into the vessel wall causing arteriosclerosis. Arteriosclerosis is associated with the high risk of heart attack and stroke.

During starvation, the triglycerides, are taken to the liver from the fat depots and broken into fatty acids and glycerol. The fatty acids are further broken into short chain compounds called **ketones**. The ketones are transported in the circulation and carried to the cells of the body wherein they are burned to produce energy. This happens when the carbohydrates consumed by the person do not fulfill the energy requirements of the body. This also happens when in a diabetic, due to the lack of insulin, glucose cannot be utilized and the patient depends on fats to fulfill his energy requirements. As more triglycerides need to be transported in circulation in uncontrolled diabetes, the level of triglycerides and hence LDL cholesterol is high.

In type 1diabetes where there is absolute lack of insulin, the body heavily depends on ketones for its energy needs often resulting in ketosis (high levels of ketones in the blood) and ketonuria (presence of ketones in urine). Whenever the level of ketone in blood becomes high, ketones spill or overflow into urine resulting in ketonuria.

Dr. Christie M. Ballantyne, director of the Center for Cardiovascular Protection at Baylor College of Medicine has recommended that LDL levels should not exceed **100 mgs%**. This is especially for those who are at high risk of developing heart attack such as diabetics.

Table 4.4 Showing normal and abnormal levels of various fats in the blood.

Range	Total Blood Cholesterol (mgs%)	HDL Cholesterol (mgs%)	LDL Cholesterol (mgs%)	Triglycerides (mgs%)
Normal	180	35 or higher	130	150-200
Borderline High	180-240	–	130-160	200-400
High	>240	–	>160	–
Normal Range: Total Lipids – 400-1000 mgs%				

Chapter 5

Human Physiology: Normal Body Functions

It is crucial to imbibe the normal so as to comprehend the abnormal.

This chapter is devoted to the normal functioning of the human system. It does not invade the intricate details but merely skirmishes the surface. Only a segment of human physiology that details how the cells of the body derive energy from the food we eat and perform myriads of functions to sustain life is mentioned.

Human body is made up of millions of cells. Cells are like tiny bricks or akin to building blocks in lego sets, which assemble to form the various systems in the human body. Cells are of several types and collect together to form various organs and structures (tissues), e.g. heart, lungs, liver and muscles. The cells get specialized to form different organs and organ systems to perform specialized functions.

The human physiology details how the cells of the body derive energy from the food we eat and perform myriad of functions to sustain life.

The food that we eat gives energy to the cells to execute mechanical, chemical and electrical activities of the body. The mechanical functions include physical activities running, walking, eating, talking, etc. The chemical functions include the synthesis of digestive juices, the formation of hormones such as sex hormones for reproductive activity, secretion of growth hormone for body growth and many more. The electrical impulses are generated in nerve cells in brain and spinal cord and then transmitted through the nerves. For example, when brain commands the leg muscles to run, the signal travels along the nerves from the brain to the legs, the nerves conducting the electrical impulse.

The cells of the body need energy to perform various functions. Each cell in the body absorbs glucose and oxygen from the blood and within the cell glucose is broken down to release energy.

The energy is released by the burning of glucose with the help of oxygen. The oxygen comes through breathing and enters the blood circulation and body system. The three main constituents of food, carbohydrates, fats and proteins are used as the burning fuel to provide energy. Carbohydrate is by far the most important source of energy. The human body undertakes a network of reactions to achieve this end. When carbohydrates are broken down, glucose is released, which is the principal substance involved in the intricate set of chemical reactions to liberate energy.

Table 5.1: The approximate energy value of three main food.

Food Type (1 gm)	Energy Content (KJ)
Carbohydrates	17
Fats	38
Proteins	20

Digestion of Food we Eat

The food we eat is chewed in the mouth with the help of saliva. It then trickles down the food pipe, which is present in the middle of chest behind the windpipe. From the food pipe, the food enters the stomach, which lies beneath the diaphragm-a muscular partition that separates the chest from the abdomen. (The trunk of the body is divided into two compartments, the upper chest and the lower abdomen).

The food is mixed in the stomach with stomach juices called **gastric** juice. It is churned to form a thin gruel over a period of about three hours. It is then gradually squeezed into the first part of the intestine (gut). Bile is a green colored fluid, which is formed in the liver and stored in the gallbladder. Bile and digestive juices from the pancreas pour through a duct into this portion of the intestines. The gruel is further changed into a thin fluid and food constituents are broken into simple compounds. In the course of digestion, all carbohydrates including starch are changed into monosaccharides or disaccharides. The monosaccharides thus formed are mostly glucose and fructose, a simple sugar found in fruits. The fats are split into fatty acids and glycerol and proteins into amino acids.

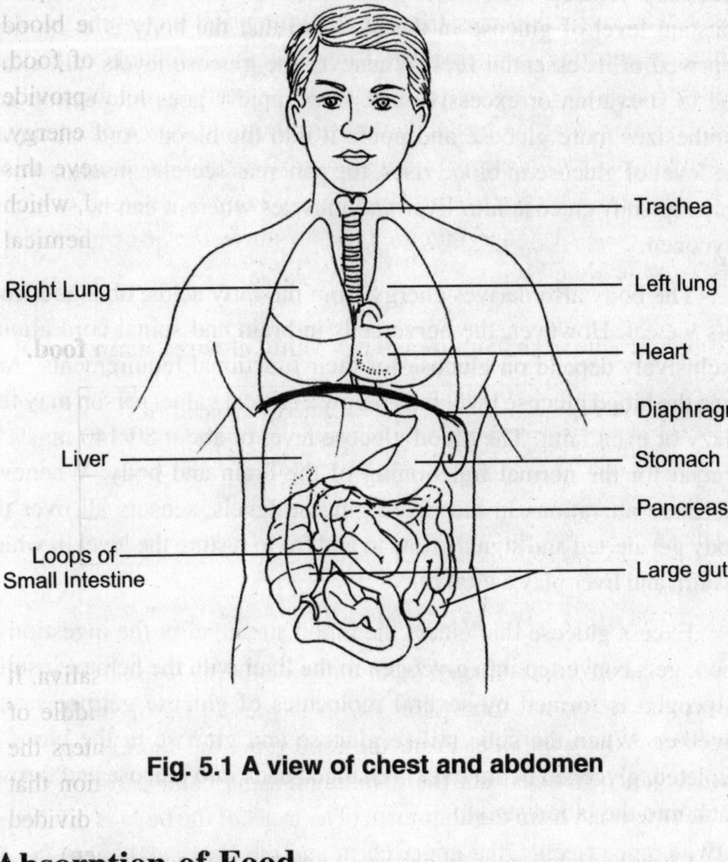

Fig. 5.1 A view of chest and abdomen

Absorption of Food

These tiny simple food molecules (compounds) are slowly absorbed from the intestinal tract and they enter the blood stream and are taken to the liver. The liver is the main workshop, which handles food constituents.

Liver can also form glucose from the food constituents brought to it, either by splitting or conversion. For example, it can convert fructose into glucose. Glucose, thus formed, re-enters the blood from the liver, from where it is picked up by the cells. Moving glucose into the cells is a complex body function. Insulin, a hormone, secreted by the pancreas, facilitates the passage of glucose into the cells where it is burned by the cells to release energy. Also, an optimum glucose level in the blood is necessary to keep cells from starving. Liver and insulin maintain a constant level of glucose in the blood so that the body is at no time deprived of its essential fuel. Whenever the glucose levels fall, either due to starvation or excessive use, liver rapidly goes into action and synthesizes more glucose and pours it into the blood. And whenever the level of glucose in blood rises, the pancreas secretes insulin, which helps to shift glucose into liver and muscles where it can be stored as glycogen.

The body also derives energy from the fatty acids, obtained from fats we eat. However, the nerve cells in brain and spinal cord almost exclusively depend on glucose for their functional requirements. Any time the blood glucose level falls below a critical value, person may feel dizzy or even faint. The blood glucose level of about 80-140 mgs% is crucial for the normal functioning of the brain and body. Whenever there are alterations in the blood glucose levels, sensors all over the body get alerted and signals flow to and fro to restore the level in which insulin and liver play a vital role.

Excess glucose that enters the blood stream after the ingestion of food, gets converted into glycogen in the liver with the help of insulin. Glycogen is formed by several molecules of glucose getting strung together. When the cells utilize glucose and glucose in the blood is depleted, glycogen in the liver is changed back into glucose and thrown back into the blood stream.

Carbohydrates eaten in excess of energy requirement of the body, are changed into fat. Fat is the **energy store** of the body. Glycogen is the **short-term storage** form of food and fat is the **long term storage** form. At the times of deprivation and starvation, body falls on its fat stores to fulfill its need.

Maintenance of Internal Milieu

As stated by *Claude Bernard*–the internal milieu is kept in a steady state. It is imperative for the viability of the cells that the internal environment is maintained in a steady state. The body is endowed with the in-built mechanism to do so. For instance in cold weather, the metabolic rate goes up, and more heat is generated so as to maintain body temperature. The reverse happens in warm weather. Be it the body temperature, blood oxygen or blood glucose levels, any shift in the normal range triggers a set of reactions that put in operations adequate measures to make necessary adjustments. This ensures the restoration of the internal environment to its original state.

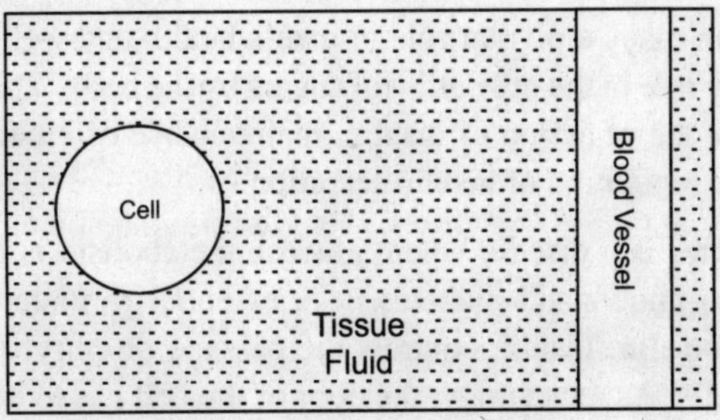

Fig. 5.2 The internal milieu/environment

Chapter 6

INSULIN AND ITS MODE OF ACTION

In the previous chapters, we explored the major constituents of food, how the food we eat is digested and absorbed from the intestine, taken to the liver, changed into glucose and made available to cells for the energy requirement and performance of various functions.

Insulin plays a pivotal role in man's health and well-being. It plays a key role in the utilisation of sugars by the body. This chapter explains mode of action of insulin, maintenance of blood glucose levels, and regulation of insulin secretion.

Diabetes is a disease where glucose metabolism is deranged. In order to understand diabetes, it is essential to understand the action of insulin. Insulin controls the passage or entry of glucose into the cells. As an analogy, the door of the cell has to be opened. The handle of the door has to be unlocked and turned. Insulin fits as a key into the lock, turns the handle and opens the door for glucose to enter.

Insulin

The discovery of insulin was a revolution. It laid the foundation for the advance in the understanding, treatment and prevention of diabetes. Pancreas** is a large endocrine gland* present in the upper part of the abdomen behind the stomach. It has head, body and tail. Scattered in the pancreas, are clusters of cells called the **islets of langerhans,** after the name of a German pathologist, Paul Langerhans, who first described these cells. Pancreas has more than a million clusters of these islets of langerhans. There are more islets located in the tail of the pancreas as compared to the body and head. Within these islets are cells called **b cells**, which form and store insulin. The insulin gets secreted into the blood directly.

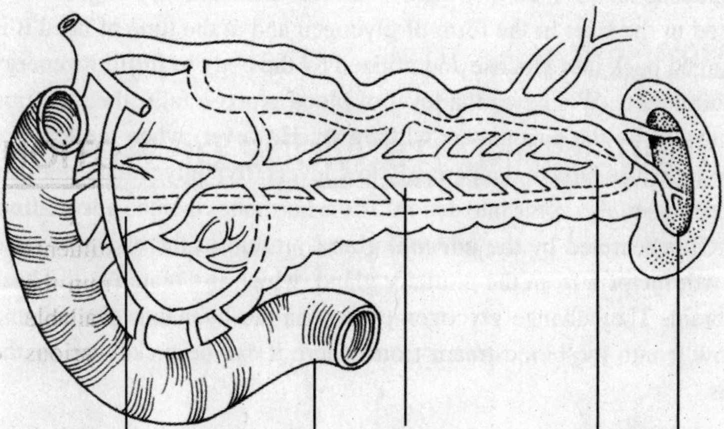

Fig. 6.1 Pancreas and Spleen

Mechanism of Insulin Secretion

The formation and secretion of the quantity of insulin is directly proportional to the level of glucose in the blood in normal persons. This is a very finely tuned and monitored mechanism that maintains the optimum level of glucose in the blood. Whenever the blood glucose level rises, insulin is secreted and it helps to bring down the glucose level and whenever the level of glucose falls, insulin is withdrawn from the circulation. When the level of glucose rises in the blood, insulin brings it down. This is achieved in two ways, one by transferring **glucose from the blood** into the body cells and secondly by converting glucose into glycogen within the liver cells and the skeletal muscle (voluntary muscles) cells. Insulin binds to receptors present on tissue cells, which facilitates entry of glucose into the cells. These receptors are like locks into which insulin fits as key opens the door through which glucose gains entry into the cell. An exception to this occurs in the brain cells and red blood cells, which imbibe glucose without the help of receptors. In the liver, glycogen store is a reserve that body falls upon in the time of need.

After a meal, the food is digested in the intestine and a large amount of glucose is absorbed into the blood. This extra amount of glucose is stored in the liver in the form of glycogen and at the time of need it is changed back into glucose and utilized by the body to fulfill its energy requirements. Whenever the level of blood glucose falls, the secretion of insulin by the pancreas is withdrawn. However, when the level of blood glucose falls to dangerously low levels (hypoglycemia) other set of hormones also come into action. These hormones include **adrenaline**, which is secreted by the **adrenal gland** present in the abdomen; and growth factor 1 from the pituitary gland, which is situated at the base of brain. They change glycogen present in the liver into glucose and throw it into the bloodstream from where it can be picked up by the cells.

The cells of the body derive their energy from the metabolism of glucose, which means utilization of glucose including its burning with the help of oxygen. The glycogen store in the muscle cells is broken into glucose and utilized during physical activity.

Normally, the islets of Langerhans maintain a perfect balance and monitor blood glucose levels by releasing appropriate amount of insulin at any given moment of time. In diabetes, this balance breaks down.

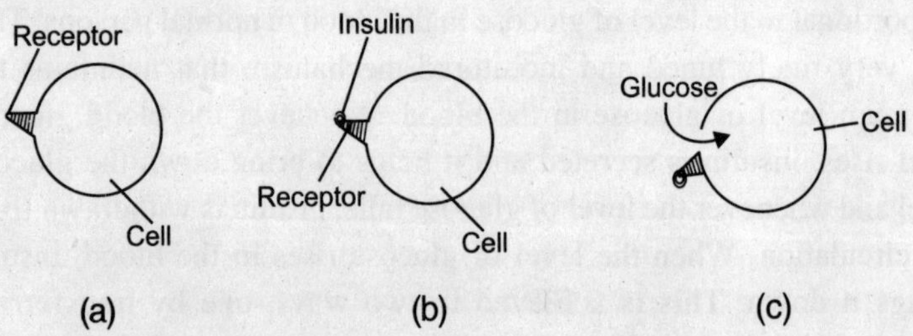

(a) Shows cell with receptor.
(b) Shows insulin linked to cell receptor.
(c) Link of insulin to receptor facilitates glucose entry into cell. Defect in link causes insulin resistence.

Fig. 6.2 Diagrammatic representation of action of Insulin

Role of Glucagons in Glucose Level Maintenance

Besides beta cells, there are alpha cells in the islets of Langerhans. The alpha cells secrete a hormone called **glucagon**. This hormone plays a role opposite to that of insulin. It tends to increase blood glucose levels. It does so by stimulating the liver to change glycogen into glucose and throw it into the bloodstream. It comes into action in hypoglycemia along with adrenaline. It also helps to maintain the normal equilibrium of blood glucose along with insulin and liver. Thus pancreas, by releasing calibrated amounts of insulin and glucagon masterminds healthy blood glucose levels and prevents dramatic swings in blood-sugar levels. Insulin promotes growth and multiplication of cells, besides regulating metabolism. Body also derives energy from fatty acids.

Diagrammatic representation of glucose circulation

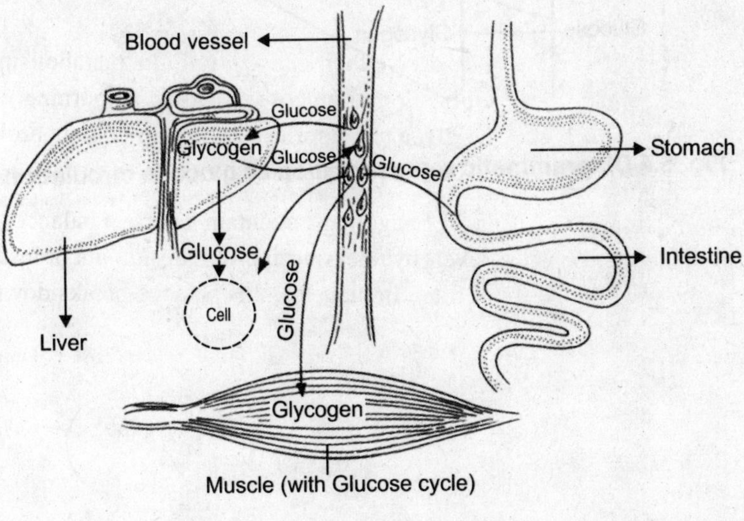

Fig. 6.3 Glucose cycle inside body

This depicts the absorption of glucose from the G-I tract into blood stream from which it is taken to the liver and muscle where it gets stored in the form of glycogen. The muscles use glycogen to derive energy during exercise. The glycogen stores in the liver are available for the energy needs of the whole body.

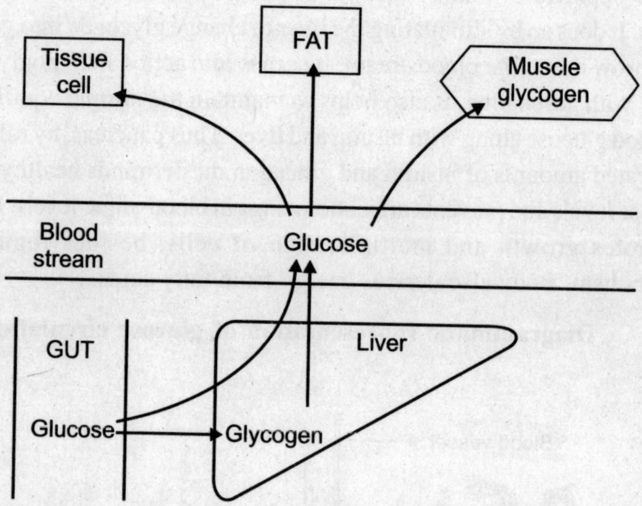

Fig. 6.4 Diagrammatic representation of glucose circulation.

---

* Gland is a structure (organ) in the body that makes substances, for example mammary glands make milk, sweat glands secrete sweat. Glands that pour their secretions into ducts are called exocrine glands, while those glands that pour their secretions into the blood stream are called endocrine glands.

** Pancreas is unique as it performs both endocrine and exocrine functions. It secretes insulin, which enters the bloodstream directly (endocrine function) and secretes digestive juices, which enter the intestine through ducts (exocrine function).

PART - II

Definition, Etiology & Complications

Chapter 7

SYMPTOMS OF DIABETES

The awareness of diabetes is exceedingly low as majority of people are not familiar with the presenting features of the disease. This chapter describes the various modes of presentation of diabetes. The association of hypertension and obesity with the diabetes is also discussed in this chapter.

I have an incident to narrate here. Long back, my husband and I were on a holiday trip in Europe. My husband drank lot of beer during the trip and to my annoyance also went to the toilet very frequently. I had to shell out money for the beer as well as his frequent visits to the toilet. At that time, it did not strike us as to what was happening. On our return home, we noticed that he had started losing weight, rather fast. Then we realized that something had gone wrong and got his blood sugar tested and it turned out to be 600 mg%.

Symptoms of Diabetes

Often symptoms are ignored for quite sometime. A person may feel hungry all the time and have uncontrolled desire to eat. He may pass urine more often and may have to get up several times during night to void urine. Sometimes, there are visual disturbances such as blurring of vision or double vision. At times there is severe pain radiating in the thighs like sciatica, or numbness or tingling in feet. The major symptoms of diabetes should be kept in mind and never to be ignored are represented in following figure:

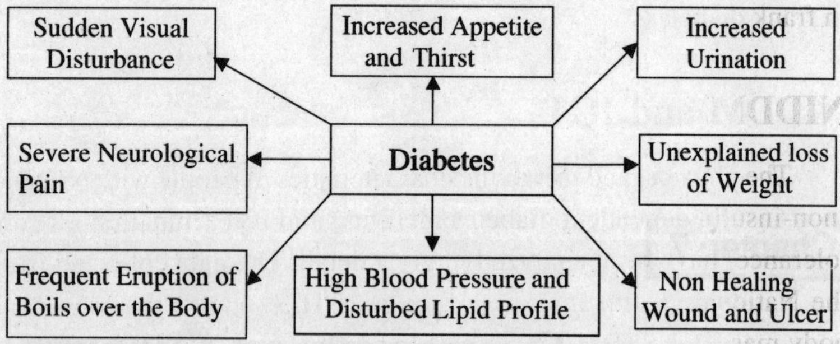

Fig. 7.1 Major symptoms of diabetes

Type 1diabetes

Type 1diabetes is also referred to as **Insulin Dependent Diabetes.** It usually occurs in people under 30 years of age but may also appear at any age. Symptoms often come on suddenly and severly. In brief, patients with type 1diabetes present more dramatically and have polyuria (increased frequency of urination), polydipsia (increased thirst), polyphagia (increased hunger) and loss of weight.

Type 2diabetes

Type 2diabetes is also known as **non-insulin dependent diabetes.** It usually occurs in people over 40 years. It develops when insulin is not able to work properly. This is called **insulin resistance**. Patients with type 2diabetes may or may not have the above symptoms and tend to have more obscure presentation. They may simply feel fatigue, blurring of vision, tingling or numbness in hands or feet. Sometimes a non-healing wound, or itching of skin or vaginites may be the first sign. Even hypertension (high blood pressure) or heart attack may be the first sign of this serious disease.

Impaired Glucose Tolerance

It is a kind of pre-diabetic phase. Here, the person is unable to handle glucose as effectively as a normal individual. The fasting blood glucose level remains higher than in a normal person but not as high as in frank diabetes.

NIDDM and IGT

The physical and metabolic characteristics of people with NIDDM (non-insulin dependent diabetes mellitus) and IGT (impaired glucose tolerance) have been analyzed in great detail. The data collected from the National Health Interview Survey (NHIS) shows that the mean body mass index (BMI) is highest in persons with NIDDM, followed by those with IGT, and then persons with normal glucose tolerance. Among people with NIDDM, the frequency of obesity (BMI>30) is much higher in women, being 46.6%, than in men, being 20.9%. Thus, incidence of obesity in women with type 2diabetes is higher than in men. It has been noted that this tendency of obesity also exists in those with predisposition to diabetes as well as those with impaired glucose tolerance. The incidence of obesity is even higher in African American women being 69.5%. Central obesity (abdominal obesity) is also more evident in persons with NIDDM and IGT as compared to normal persons. Mean blood pressure levels are also higher in persons with NIDDM and IGT as compared to normal individuals. Hypertension (blood pressure>160/95 mm Hg) in persons in the age group 65-74 is 60% in NIDDM, 50.7% in IGT and 38.3% in persons with normal glucose tolerance.

Lipid Profile

A similar tendency is observed in lipid profile. The levels of total cholesterol, LDL cholesterol and triglycerides are higher in persons with NIDDM and IGT as compared to persons with normal glucose tolerance. The level of HDL cholesterol, which is the healthy cholesterol, is lower in persons with NIDDM and IGT and higher in individuals with normal glucose tolerance.

Chapter 8

TYPES OF DIABETES

What is diabetes mellitus and what are its different variants? What is the role of heredity in various types of diabetes? What is insulin resistance? What does it imply and is there anything we can do about it? All this is touched upon in the following pages. The role of immunity is also discussed. The differences between the two main types of diabetes, type 1 and type 2 are also outlined.

Diabetes mellitus (DM) is a disorder characterized by hyperglycemia meaning high blood glucose levels, due to the complete or relative deficiency of insulin or insensitivity of the tissues to circulating insulin. Due to the lack of insulin, cells of the body fail to metabolize (utilize) glucose, as a result of which, the glucose remains high in the blood. Thus, diabetes mellitus has three main characteristics.

1. **Failure of glucose to pass from blood into cells**, either due to the lack of insulin or *insulin resistance. As discussed in previous chapters, insulin unlocks the door on cells allowing glucose to flow into the cells. When there is lack of insulin, this function is impaired. This is true in type 1diabetes but not in all cases of type 2. In type 2diabetes, often the insulin key is unable to fit into the lock on the cell and open the door. This is referred to as insulin resistance. Thus, even when there is adequate amount of insulin available in the body it is unable to operate, as the key and lock mechanism gets mismatched.
2. As a result, glucose unable to flow into the cells, remains high in the blood,
3. The cells continue to starve due to the unavailability of glucose.

Glucose is the sugar required to produce energy in the body. In a normal person, insulin regulates blood glucose levels. Whenever blood glucose level rises, more insulin is secreted; this brings the level down, and vice versa. This fine tuning gets deranged in DM. Normal fasting blood glucose, which is measured **after 8 hours** of fasting, as a routine early in the morning is < 110 mgs %. A reading between 110 mgs % and 126 mgs% is considered **impaired glucose tolerance (IGT)** and a **level above 126 mgs%** is diagnosed as DM. The blood glucose level measured **2 hours after** glucose load or proper meal is < 140 mgs % in normal cases, between 140 mgs % and 199 mgs % in impaired glucose tolerance and >200 mgs % in Diabetes. Blood glucose levels can be expressed in mgs % *i.e.* milligrams per deciliter of blood and also as mmol/liter. To convert mg/dl into millimoles/l multiply mgs by 0.055 and to convert mmol/l into mgs/dl multiply mmol by 18.01.

Table 8.1 Showing few equivalents between mg per dl and millimoles/l.

50 mg/dl	2.8 mmol/l
100 mg/dl	5.6 mmol/l
150 mg/dl	8.3 mmol/l
200 mg/dl	11.1 mmol/l

Four major types of diabetes have been defined by the WHO (World Health Organization) and NDDG (National Diabetic Data Group). These are IDDM (insulin dependent diabetes mellitus), NIDDM (non-insulin dependent diabetes), GDM (gestational diabetes mellitus) and others that are secondary to other diseases. There are however two common or conventional types.

Type 1 DM, IDDM (Insulin Dependent Diabetes Mellitus)

In this type, there is almost total deficiency of insulin. It comprises of about 10% of all types of diabetes cases. It manifests in the juvenile age group, but can occur at any age. It is occasionally seen in non-obese adults. It usually occurs below the age of 30. In this type, the patient requires insulin from external source for the control of DM, as his pancreas is unable to produce insulin. There is genetic predisposition and environmental influence in the development of type 1DM. It is an autoimmune disorder where there is destruction of b cells of pancreas by body's own T lymphocytes.

Immune Dysfunction In Type 1diabetes

Our body is endowed with its own immune system or defense system. Like any military, our system has its range of weapons. There are white blood cells (present in blood), which are akin to guns, and antibodies, which are akin to bullets/missiles. When any germ enters our body, our defense system takes its print and manufactures antibodies (bullets) specific to the print to kill the invading germ. Normally, the body does not form antibodies against its own cells. But sometimes this function gets haywire. In this variant of diabetes, there is an autoimmune disorder*** wherein the patient develops antibodies against his own insulin and pancreatic beta islet cells.

Antibodies are substances circulating in the blood, which are protein in nature, and produced by the immune system (defense system) of the body. Antibodies are generated as part of the body defense mechanism, in response to antigens, which under normal circumstances are foreign proteins or protein complexes. In other words, antibodies are like missiles that are produced by the body's defense system (immune system) to attack foreign invaders (antigens). These antibodies damage or inactivate the antigen against which they have been produced. For example, when bacteria infect a person, which is a foreign invader, the human body regards it as an alien. And as part of it's complicated defense arsenal it forms antibodies to inactivate the bacterial proteins, which are known as antigens. Under normal conditions, the human body does not produce antibodies against its own cells and tissues. But in an autoimmune disorder, the immune system goes haywire and it's aberrant activity results in the formation of antibodies against its own body cells. It could also be possible that the pancreatic cell surface antigens, by which the immune system recognizes the cells as self, get altered and defy recognition.

Every cell in the body has surface markers, a kind of ID by which the cells are recognized as self or own as against foreign cells such as viruses. If the ID of the cell gets spoiled or damaged or altered, the cell will be regarded as foreign and killed. Thus, in type 1diabetes there is immune dysfunction. The immune system starts forming antibodies against its own pancreatic beta cells, the cells that manufacture insulin. With the inactivation of pancreatic beta cells, the production of insulin is greatly reduced and the patient is totally dependent on insulin from external source for his metabolic needs. It has been shown that 80-

90% of the beta cells get destroyed before diabetes becomes manifest. Evidence in favor of the autoimmune mechanism in the development of type 1DM, is the presence of specific antibodies against pancreatic beta cells in the patient's blood.

Genetic Control of Type 1diabetes

There is a very strong genetic predisposition and association with HLA-DR3 or HLA-DR4** (gene code) in type 1DM. Those individuals who inherit this genetic code are highly vulnerable to type 1diabetes. These genetic codes also determine the activity of T lymphocytes. **T lymphocytes are a class of white blood cells, which play an important role in the regulation of immune response of the body.** T lymphocytes are among the body's vast arsenal required to produce chemicals (among them antibodies) to fight foreign invaders and disease germs. They are like guns that fire bullets (antibodies) to kill viruses and bacteria. The association of Type 1diabetes with the genetic code dealing with the defense mechanisms`indicate a strong link between heredity, immunity and type 1 DM. Often a viral infection, such as mumps or German measles, precipitates the autoimmune process. It was felt that vaccination might help to decrease the incidence of this type of diabetes. However, in Finland where type 1diabetes is prevalent, vaccination against viruses did not make any significant difference. Ketosis and keturia, which means the presence of ketone bodies in blood and urine respectively, a life threatening condition, can occur in this type of diabetes.

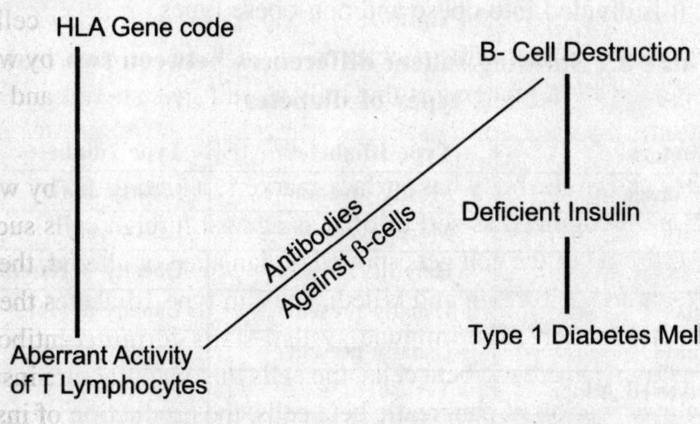

Fig. 8.1 Heredity-immunity-type 1diabetes

Another advance in this direction has been the discovery of **Tap 1** and **Tap 2** genes. These genes control the immune defense of cells. These genes have been found to influence the interaction of cell surface antigens and the immune system. In an experimental research, when healthy Tap genes were inserted into the diabetic cells, 40% of the cells became recognizable as 'self' by the immune system.

Type 2 DM or NIDDM (Non-Insulin Dependent Diabetes Mellitus)

Although, environmental factors, such as sedentary life style plays an important role in the genesis of type 2 DM, genetic factors are even more important. In this type, patient does not require external source of insulin to control his diabetes in the early stages. It is a heterogenous group, predominantly found in adults over the age of 40, but can occur in younger individuals, especially in Native Americans. The main type of NIDDM, associated with insulin resistance and beta cell failure may also comprise several entities, both genetic and non-genetic.

All characters in our body are hereditary, passing from parents to offspring by virtue of genes. **The genes control all functions in the body. Some functions are controlled by the single gene while others are under the influence of several genes.** Thus, if 5 genes control a process, then a defect in any one of the 5 genes will cause disease. Hence, a disease may have several genetic causes.

Type 2diabetes is one such example and is further divided into several types, based on the genetic defects and forms a heterogeneous group. It is divided into obese and non-obese types.

Table 8.2 Showing salient differences between two main types of diabetes

Parameters	Type 1diabetes	Type 2diabetes
Age of onset	Mostly juvenile	Mostly adult
Intensity	More severe	Less severe
Cause	Heredity	Obesity + Heredity
Ketosis	Usually present	Usually absent
Ketonuria	Usually present	Usually absent
Linked to HLA loci	Yes	No
Dependence on insulin	Absolute dependence on insulin	May or may not require insulin

Insulin Resistance

In more than 90% of patients of type 2diabetes, there is evidence of insulin resistance. In this condition, the tissues of the body especially liver, muscle and fat require extra insulin to maintain normal glycemic control as compared to normal persons. As the tissues fail to respond to normal levels of insulin and fail to use the glucose present in blood, the level of glucose rises. In response to the high level of glucose, there is increased outpouring of insulin by the pancreas. Insulin resistance in the periphery results in increased production of insulin by the pancreas. This results in high levels of insulin in the blood.

Insulin resistance can occur even before diabetes becomes manifest. In the early phases, the pancreas secretes extra insulin to compensate for this insulin resistance, so that blood glucose levels remain within normal limits. Later, pancreas fails to keep up with this extra demand and the blood glucose goes up and type 2diabetes becomes manifest. It is now believed that any degree of insulin resistance increases a person's risk of heart disease. Drugs like **actos** and **avandia** act primarily by making muscle and fat tissues more responsive to insulin, so that they use glucose more effectively and readily and bring down the blood glucose levels. **Targretin** is a drug on trial and it has been found to lower insulin resistance.

Research has shown that reduced mitochondrial activity in the cells in adults translate to higher levels of intercellular lipid which causes insulin resistance.

Insulin Resistance in Type 2 DM

In NIDDM, there is often insulin resistance. Two defects characterize this disease, one is failure of tissue cells to respond to insulin (insulin resistance) and second failure of pancreatic cells to produce adequate amount of insulin in face of hyperglycemia. As cells fail to respond to insulin, the beta cells of pancreas produce more and more insulin to overcome resistance. At this stage, the level of insulin in blood is higher than normal, although ineffective. However, after some time the pancreatic cells get exhausted and start failing. With beta cell failure, the level of insulin starts falling.

This main form of NIDDM, associated with insulin resistance and beta cell failure, may also comprise several etiologic entities, both genetic and non-genetic. Many rare genetic syndromes are associated with the glucose intolerance. Both insulin resistance (which means failure of insulin action to transport glucose from the circulation into the cells) and beta cell failure (which means lack of production of adequate amount of insulin) have multiple genetic causes and result in many types of NIDDM. Beta cell failure may be secondary to insulin resistance, may be concurrent with or may even precede it. It is estimated that 50% of beta cell dysfunction is present at the time of diagnosis and continues to increase with the passing time.

There is a strong familial and genetic predisposition. It has been seen that in identical twins, if one of the twins develops diabetes, the other will also have it.

Type 2diabetes is further divided into obese and non-obese variants. Obesity is often linked to insulin resistance.

Obesity-Insulin Resistance Type 2diabetes

In this class of DM, the cells of the body tissues show decreased response to insulin present in the circulation. Even when adequate amount of insulin is available, the cells fail to respond to it and do not get glucose for their energy needs. The cells continue to starve even when the levels of glucose in the blood are high. The pancreas also reveals decrease responsiveness to variations in the glucose levels in the blood. Even when the level of glucose is high, with beta cell failure, the pancreas fails to secrete insulin to bring the level down. Both these defects, insulin resistance and beta cell failure, are aggravated by abdominal-visceral obesity. Abdominal-visceral obesity means excessive amount of fat present inside the abdomen.

PC-1 Protein in Type 2diabetes

This compound is more prevalent in people with type 2 diabetics than non-diabetics. The over production of this substance is genetically determined. It is believed to interfere with the normal functioning of insulin receptors.

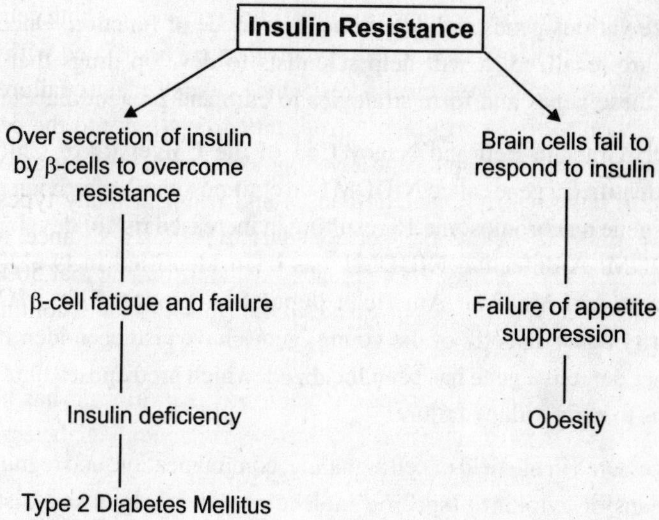

Fig. 8.2 Obesity-Insulin Resistance-b Cell failure-type 2diabetes

Type 1diabetes is More Severe than Type 2

Type 2 also differs from type 1 in that ketosis and ketonuria usually do not occur in this. The type 2 variant is also not linked to HLA genes, nor is there any autoimmune reaction in the body. However, type 2 is more common than type 1. About 90% of the diabetic patients belong to type 2 category.

Both type 1 and type 2 DM are complex diseases, which arise from defective genes. A number of genes are involved in the formation, secretion and utilization of insulin and any subtle variation in the gene results in defective gene. These abnormal genes interact with other genes and the environment. In type 1 DM, the susceptible gene reacts to environmental triggers such as viruses. In type 2 DM, the genes react to external influences like obesity and inactivity, resulting in the development of diabetes or a greater risk of getting the disease.

Genetic Research on Diabetes Mellitus

An International Type 2DM Genetic Linkage Consortium has been formed to help researchers to combine their individual findings and localize various genes and determine their mode of function. Once the genes are localized, it will help scientists to develop drugs that will target these genes and form strategies to cure and prevent diabetes.

Dr. Graenne Bell and Nancy Cox of the University of Chicago have identified a gene called NIDDM1 on chromosome 2, which interacts with a gene on chromosome 15 resulting in increased risk of developing type 2DM. A defective NIDDM1 has been identified in two North European and Mexican American population groups. Five **MODY** (maturity onset diabetes of the young) genes have also been identified. Another defective gene has been localized, which predisposes the Pima Indians to early kidney failure.

Research in the field of cell signaling, communication, and regulation by means of cytokines (specific molecules) have helped scientists to understand the working of the immune system and what goes wrong in autoimmune disorders such as type 1diabetes. This is also shedding light on insulin resistance, which precedes type 2diabetes.

Nuclear hormone receptors**** regulate gene expression. There are certain receptors in the brain. When insulin acts on these receptors, appetite is suppressed. In case insulin is not taken up by the receptors in the brain, there is failure of appetite-suppressing effect. Researchers at Harvard University's Joslin Diabetes Center found that without these brain receptors mice, become obese and insulin resistant. These reports reinforce that a complex network of molecular signals and feedback loops involving brain and other tissues are key to unraveling the mystery of obesity and insulin resistance that precedes type 2diabetes. Besides these two main types of diabetes, there are some less common forms of diabetes also.

GDM (Gestational Diabetes Mellitus)

This type of diabetes develops during pregnancy. The incidence among pregnant women is about 3-5%. Such subjects revert to normal when pregnancy ends. However, 35-50% of such women progress to non-insulin dependent diabetes mellitus later in life, especially if they are overweight. GDM is also associated with obesity, positive family history and older age. Investigators believe that same genetic defects are present in these individuals as in type 2DM.

The prevalence of congenital birth defects in infants born of diabetic mothers is about 10%. About 3% to 5% of pregnancies in diabetic women result in the death of the newborn. Premature births, complications at the time of delivery and risks to newborn infant can develop.

This variant may remain asymptomatic or patient may develop symptoms similar to other types of diabetes. A regular blood sugar test is imperative especially in high-risk women. The cause of this variant of diabetes is not fully understood. Some scientists believe that unrecognized diabetes is already present in such cases. The weight gain and hormonal alterations simply precipitate and unmask the disease.

Other forms of Diabetes (Secondary Diabetes)

The prevalence of other variants of DM is 1-2% of the total incidence of this disease. These variants are listed below.

1. There is reduction of beta cell mass in the pancreas in certain conditions e.g. in malignant disease of the pancreas and surgical removal of the pancreas. Also, in pancreatites, an inflammatory disease of the pancreas, the functional beta cell mass is destroyed. **Pancreatites** is fairly common in South India. Secondary diabetes is common in children due to severe protein malnutrition in the third world countries like India, Indonesia and Jamaica.

   In other cases of secondary diabetes, there is relative deficiency of insulin due to the over production of other group of hormones, which are antagonistic to insulin.
2. Chemical agents toxic to the beta cells of the pancreas, as pentamidine and vacor, similarly reduce the beta cell mass.
3. Genetic defects in a -cell function.
4. MODY (maturity onset diabetes of the young) 1, 2, 3, 4, 5.
5. Genetic defects in insulin function.
6. Exocrine pancreatic diseases e.g. pancreatitis, carcinoma, cystic fibrosis.

7. Drug / chemical-induced.
8. Infections e.g. congenital rubella, CMV.
9. Drugs that increase blood sugar levels. For example, Chlorthalidone, Diazoxide, Furosemide, Epinephrine, Estrogen, Nicotinic acid, Phenytoin, Thyroid preparations, Thiazide, Glucagon, Caffeine and Morphine.
10. Drugs that lower blood sugar levels. For example, Alcohol, Insulin, Beta-blockers, Anabolic steroids, Fenfluramine, Salicylates and Phenobarbital.

---

* Insulin Resistance. Insulin attaches itself to receptors present on cell surface and facilitates the flow of glucose into the cell. A defect in insulin-receptor link hinders this function resulting in insulin resistance.

** HLA-DR3 and HLA-DR4. The human genome is a lengthy sequence of genes. They have a specific nomenclature. HLA-DR3 and 4 are names of genes that are associated with body's immune (defense) system and control body's immune response and are associated with tissue matching and compatibility.

*** Autoimmune disorder. The body's defense system (immune system) starts manufacturing missiles (antibodies) against its own cells and destroys them.

**** Receptors are structures present on cell surface. They link to other molecules and set in motion a cycle of reactions. For example certain brain receptors link to insulin and set a cycle in motion, which suppresses appetite. When these receptors are absent or defective, appetite is not suppressed and person has tendency to eat more and become obese

Chapter 9

DIAGNOSIS AND MANAGEMENT OF DIABETES

How to know that you have diabetes and how to be absolutely sure that it is not something else? This chapter pertains to WHO diagnostic criteria, and how to monitor the blood sugar levels? What is the significance of urine examination and when and why to do these tests? Some other conditions associated with high blood glucose levels are also tabulated.

Laboratory Tests for Diagnosis of Diabetes

In a person suspected to be suffering from diabetes, diagnosis can be established by the blood tests and urine analysis.

Blood Glucose Test

The criterion for confirmation of diabetes is the estimation of blood glucose levels. A fasting plasma glucose level of 126 mg% or more, on more than one occasion helps to establish the diagnosis of diabetes. Normal fasting glucose level is up to 110 mg%. If the fasting plasma glucose level is borderline than a standardized oral glucose tolerance test may be done, keeping in mind the age factor.

Impaired Glucose Tolerance (IGT) is a class that encompasses those persons whose glucose tolerance is in between normal and diabetic patients. They constitute about 11% of the adults and are at higher risk of developing **frank diabetes**. Here, the fasting glucose level is between 110-126 mg%.

An International Expert Committee that was sponsored by the American Diabetes Association has recently made recommendations for the diagnosis, screening and testing for diabetes mellitus.

Fasting plasma glucose is the preferred test for the diagnosis and screening of DM. The committee has recommended it over oral glucose tolerance as it is cost effective, easier to perform and reproducible.

Glycosylated Haemoglobin (HbA_{1c}) Measurement

The glucose molecules present in the blood combine with haemoglobin present in the red blood cells in the blood, to form a stable compound called **glycosylated haemoglobin**. The higher the level of glucose in the blood, the higher the amount of glycosylated hemoglobin formed. Hence in diabetes, as the level of glucose is higher than normal the glycosylated haemoglobin estimates are also higher than normal. As the life of red blood cells is three months on an average, these values of HbA_{1c} also persist for three months. If the estimated level of HbA_{1c} is more than normal it indicates that the glucose level has remained high in the previous 3 months duration. Thus, these estimates reflect the level of metabolic control in diabetes over the previous three-month period. Such evaluations are important in the control and management of diabetes. The results of the DCCT (Diabetes Control Complications Trial) showed a direct relationship between HbA_{1c} values and the risk of developing chronic complications.

Fructosamine Assay

It reflects the glycemic control over the immediate previous period of 1 to 2 weeks. These two tests are a useful complement to the daily monitoring of blood glucose in achieving optimal glucose control, and should not be used as a substitute for the latter.

These tests are not recommended for the diagnosis of DM, but only for the management and control of the disease.

Table 9.1 Comparison between Haemoglobin A_{1c} and blood glucose level

Blood Parameters	Levels in Blood				
Haemoglobin A1c	5-6	5-6	6-8	8-11	11-14
Blood glucose	90-120	90-120	150-180	180-270	270-360
Control	Normal	Good	Fair	Poor	VeryPoor

Self-Monitoring of Blood Glucose Level

Glucometer

At present many types of glucometers, which are small, easy and convenient to use are available in the market. They are operated on battery and are handy and portable. With a simple finger prick by a tiny sharp lancet, blood is drawn onto a paper strip, which is then inserted into the machine. Within minutes, the blood sugar value is displayed on the screen.

Many newer models of glucometers, which have dispensed with finger pricking and paper strips, are also available.

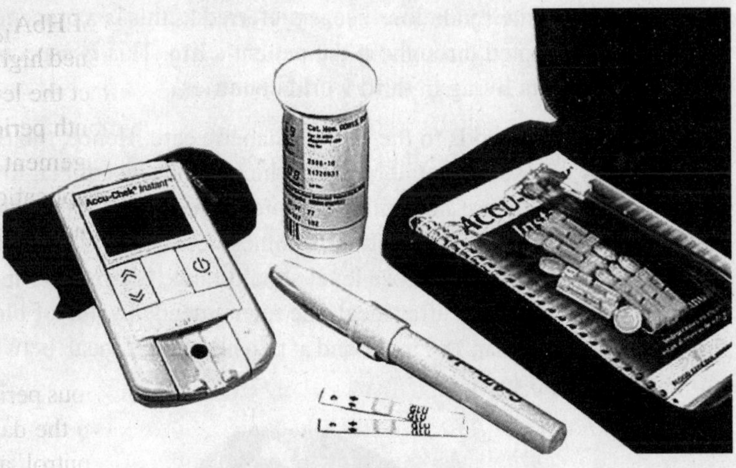

Fig. 9.1 Glucometer

Glucowatch

A newer innovation, called **glucowatch** recently approved by the FDA, is a device, which estimates glucose levels by using **sensors**. This eliminates the need to draw blood by finger pricks. This is extremely useful in children suffering from type 1diabetes, in which sugar levels need to be tested several times a day. It also works during sleep and sounds an alarm when glucose hits dangerously low or high levels-lifesaving as that happens when a child is asleep. Within minutes the blood glucose level is displayed on the screen. Such estimates help the patient to learn about his diabetic status more frequently and help to regulate his condition. Such self-estimations are essential in the regulation and management of type 1diabetes. These are also valuable in type 2diabetes.

In type 1diabetes, the blood sugar levels have to be tested several times during the day, as patient is on insulin and needs constant monitoring. In type 2, it is advisable to test blood sugar levels twice a day, after medication has been prescribed and standardized. The test should be done once fasting and then before lunch and/ or dinner. If done only once, then it is preferred to check fasting glucose level. Some individuals check once a day alternating fasting and pre lunch timing. Some authors recommend a more frequent testing of blood sugar levels, more than twice a day. The paper strips used in the machine are expensive and their judicious use is preferred as this is a procedure, which is to be adopted throughout the patient's life. This is especially true for the patients living in third world countries.

Frequent testing adds to the cost of diabetic care. Hence, the time and frequency of testing should be that, which is most beneficial to the patient. If the results are not within the prescribed limits on repeated examination, a medical consultation becomes necessary. In a diabetic patient, the fasting blood glucose level should range between 90 mg% to 120 mg%. At one hour after meal, the recommended value of blood glucose level is less than 180 mg% and at two hours after meal, between 140 mg% and 160 mg%.

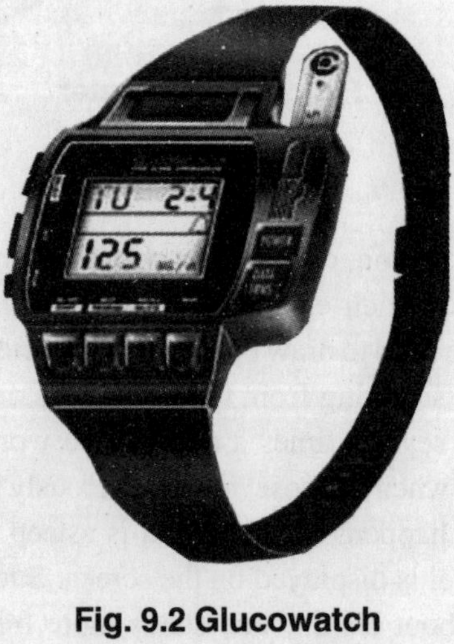

Fig. 9.2 Glucowatch

Precautions while Using Glucose Meters

Carefully follow instructions given in the manual of the Glucometer kit. While using glucose meters, certain precautions should be taken. Some important ones are listed below:

1. Use fresh glucose strips that are not discolored or have expired.
2. Periodically calibrate the meter with the control solution.
3. Keep the meter clean.
4. Periodically compare the meter results to laboratory results; the results should be within 15% of each other.
5. Replace meter batteries regularly.

A close and regular contact with the health care personal and doctor and an on-going self-education go a long way in helping the patient lead a normal life.

Urine Test for Glucose

The patient can also evaluate his diabetic status at home by testing his urine, instead of blood by the simple paper strip method marketed as Diastix. These strips for testing urinary glucose are very cheap and can be used more frequently without worrying about the cost. These can help to detect as little as 0.1% glucose in urine. The color change in the strip gives a rough estimate of the amount of glucose present in the urine. However, certain drugs especially if taken in large doses, such as, aspirin and vitamin C can interfere with the test results. However, the urine testing is becoming obsolete. The reason being results of urine tests only give a rough estimate of the blood glucose levels. In fact, sugar appears in urine only when the blood glucose **level exceeds 180 mg%** and then sugar spills into urine. Also, the urine sample being tested has collected over a period of time and gives no indication of the current status. This anomaly can be mitigated to some extent by using double voided urine sample. This method, however has become obsolete in the USA but is still prevalent in third world countries.

The advantage of urine testing is that it is cheap and if the test is positive on repeated examinations it surely indicates uncontrolled diabetes mellitus.

But urine ketone testing still remains an important procedure in patients with type 1 DM and patients with gestational diabetes. Self-monitoring of blood glucose levels is as important as planning the meals, the daily office activity, the daily medication and exercise. Keeping accurate records of the results of blood glucose levels and daily routine helps the patient regulate his diabetes in a more scientific manner rather than depending on guesswork.

Hyperglycemia due to other Causes

There are many causes of hyperglycemia besides diabetes. These include some tumors and some non-tumorous conditions of adrenal and pituitary glands and certain disorders of the liver. These conditions should be considered in the differential diagnosis of diabetes. A number of other hormones are produced in the body, which have action opposite to that of insulin. Different glands in the body produce these hormones.

Table 9.2 Various causes of Hyperglycemia

Name of Tumor or condition	Origin of Condition	Hormone Produced
Glucagons secreting tumor	Pancreas	Glucagons with action oppo site to insulin
Cushing syndrome	Adrenal gland	Cortisone causes hyperglyce mia
Prolactin secreting tumor	Pituitary gland	Prolactin blocks insulin action
Acromegaly	Pituitary gland	Growth hormone blocks insu lin sensitivity
Pheochromocytoma	Adrenal gland	Adrenalin causes hyperglyce mia
Hyperthyroidism	Thyroid gland	Thyroxine causes glucose intol erance
Stomatostatin secreting tumor	Pancreas	Stomatostatin blocks insulin secretion by islet cells

Chapter 10

DIABETES & PREGNANCY AND DIABETES & ALCOHOL

What precautions to take and what rules to follow when diabetes is associated with pregnancy?

The perverse fascination for alcoholic drinks and relentless decline in simple living has, driven man away from nature and made him prey to many ailments. Excessive alcohol wrecks the human body, more so in a diabetic.

The most rewarding and most fulfilling experience of modern innovations is saving babies of pregnant women with diabetes. One heart-rending incident comes to my mind again and again. It occurred nearly 40 years ago, when I was posted in maternity ward as an intern. A full term diabetic woman had been admitted. It was a very precious baby, being the first, as the woman had conceived after several years of marriage. It was a premature delivery. Unfortunately, the baby died at the time of birth. The mother was devastated and the father writhed with agony.

We have come a long way through excellent medical scientific innovations. Now it is no longer the code that a diabetic woman cannot conceive a baby, as was the situation several years' back, when repeated still births and miscarriages were the order of the day. Now-a-days pregnancy can be planned, carried to full term and motherhood rejoiced.

Diabetes in Pregnant Women

The pregnancy has to be planned well before conception. Some non-diabetic women develop diabetes during pregnancy-gestational diabetes. These women require as much meticulous care during pregnancy as their diabetic companions. Rigid criteria have been established for screening gestational diabetes. Glucose tolerance tests are done to find out low and high-risk women. Depending on specific population groups, abnormal glucose tolerance occurs in 3-10% of pregnancies. Incidence of GDM (Gestational Diabetes Mellitus) is 1.5-2% in white Americans, 5-8% in Hispanics, Afro-Americans and Asians. The frequency is higher in Native Americans, going up to 15%. To detect cases of GDM screening tests are done in the first trimester. Screening tests are more pertinent in the following instances.

- Maternal age > 35 years
- Previous large baby
- Unexplained demise of previous baby
- Family history of diabetes
- Obesity
- High blood glucose levels in previous pregnancy

Precautions before Conception

Before a woman conceives, she must control her diabetes. It is recommended that HbA1c should be less than 7%. She must lose weight in case of obesity. Also, she should get examined for kidney or eye complications, as these get aggravated during pregnancy. A rigid and tight control of blood sugar has to be achieved, to create a healthy environment, for conception to occur.

Precautions for Diabetic Pregnant Woman

When a diabetic woman becomes pregnant, she has to take extra precautions while managing her diabetes. During pregnancy, high blood sugar levels can harm the mother as well as the baby she is carrying. Eye and other complications can develop or get worse if they are already present. Diabetic nephropathy advances if glycemic control is poor.

During pregnancy, oral antidiabetic drugs are contraindicated as they harm the babies and are to be avoided strictly. Drug of choice is insulin. The pregnant mother has to be fully versed with the use of insulin. The amount of insulin given is to be carefully monitored, as the nutritional demand on the mother increases as pregnancy advances and the dose of insulin has to be adjusted along with the dietary intake to maintain a steady balance. Also with the growth of placenta, there is surge of placental hormones, which induce insulin resistance. It is recommended that six meals be given during pregnancy, blood glucose levels to be checked several times during the day and hypoglycemia and hyperglycemia avoided at all costs. The glucose profile of these women should be a meticulous replication of healthy women to avoid morbidities. There is an increased tendency for hypoglycemia, which should be avoided by keeping a ready snack at hand. Exercise is a must but should never be rigorous.

Maternal morbidity is high and **hypertension** and **pre-eclampsia** take their toll. Besides miscarriage and birth defects, large babies form. Strict blood sugar control before conception and during pregnancy decreases the incidence of birth defects by 1-5 %. Uncontrolled diabetes mellitus increases birth anomalies by 4-8 fold.

To be able to control her diabetes well, woman must keep certain things in mind.

1. She must monitor her blood sugar daily and if necessary more than twice a day.
2. A daily urine examination for ketone bodies is mandatory, as pregnancy with diabetes is more predisposed to ketoacidosis.
3. Oral glucose lowering agents are not recommended during pregnancy.
4. The dose of insulin will need to be adjusted as the requirement of insulin increases during pregnancy.
5. The meal plan and the calorie requirement have to be worked out carefully so as to meet the demands of pregnancy.
6. A regular consultation with the health provider should be assured.
7. A diabetic pregnant mother must always abstain from alcohol, drugs and smoking.
8. The use of artificial sweeteners is not recommended in pregnancy.
9. A good snack must always be kept handy in case of hypoglycemia, which tends to occur more often in pregnancy.

Large Babies

Large babies, weighing as much as 4000 gms or more develop as high blood sugar in the maternal blood pass into the babies circulation and stimulate the pancreas to produce increased amount of insulin. The overactive pancreatic state, thus induced, extends into the early neonatal period causing complications. The increased secretion of insulin, in turn **changes excess sugar into fat**, which gets stored in the baby making it big and overweight. Foetal obesity develops a unique pattern of growth with deposition of excessive fat in the central abdomen and interscapular region. Foetal birth weight correlate more with postprandial blood sugar rather than fasting levels. Accelerated growth thus stimulated often extends into childhood and adulthood. Foetal overgrowth causes hypoxia resulting in defects in cardiovascular and central nervous system.

Large babies make delivery difficult and may necessitate caesarian section. Large babies may also induce pre-mature labor and are also susceptible to hypoglycemia soon after birth due to their overactive pancreas. Biophysical profile of the baby needs regular monitoring during pregnancy and the time and route of delivery carefully evaluated during the last trimester. When blood sugar levels are within normal range in the mother, normal size babies develop.

Diabetes and Alcohol

There are many contradictory views regarding the consumption of alcohol in diabetes. Some authors permit moderate intake of alcohol, not more than 2 drinks per day for men and not more than 1 drink per day for women, only when diabetes is under complete control. One drink being equivalent to 12 oz beer, 5 oz wine, or 1.5 oz of distilled spirits. Other authors recommend that smoking and drinking should be totally restricted.

These habits of drinking and smoking do not confer any benefit on the health of the individual but have definite and distinctive harmful effects. Chronic excessive **alcoholic abuse** damages the pancreas depleting its capacity to form and secrete insulin. Alcohol puts diabetes control out of gear and causes chaos in blood sugar levels. It can produce hyperglycemia as well as dangerous, life-threatening hypoglycemia. It disturbs lipid profile, raises tryglyceride levels, increases blood pressure and thereby potentiates cardiac complications. However, in the following instances patient should totally refrain from drinking.

1. In the event of pancreatitis, which is inflammation of the pancreas.
2. Kidney dysfunction.
3. Lipid disorders.
4. Complications affecting nervous system.
5. During pregnancy.
6. Overweight patients.
7. Patients given to alcoholic abuse.
8. Patients taking high doses of insulin are at risk of developing hypoglycemia and these individuals on taking alcohol further aggravate the risk.
9. Alcohol is to be strictly avoided in case of fever or any infectious disease.
10. During the recovery phase of any physical injury or trauma.

Chapter 11

PATHOGENESIS OF DIABETES

This chapter briefly describes the role of cardiovascular system in preserving the internal environment. It then goes on to elaborate the alterations that take place inside the body when a person develops diabetes. It further discusses the consequences of these changes and their role in the development of complications. This chapter also describes how the deposition of bad cholesterol or LDL into vessel walls compromises the circulation of blood and how antioxidants affect the genesis of atherosclerosis.

The human body is made up of tissues, which in turn are made up of billions of cells. The cells are basic unit of organic life. These cells are present in columns, layers and bundles while forming an organ. The cells are constantly bathed in a fluid called the **tissue fluid**. The tissue fluid separates the cells from one another and flows like a stream around them. Each cell requires food in the form of glucose, besides water and oxygen, for survival. Oxygen is needed to burn down glucose to release energy to sustain life. As cells perform their vital functions, lot of waste substance is generated. The waste also requires to be removed from the system. The cells throw their waste into the tissue fluid and receive their nutrients through the same medium.

Circulatory System

The circulatory system or cardiovascular system fulfills the basic needs of the body with the help of other organs in the body, including liver, lungs and kidneys. The circulatory system is made of heart and blood vessels. The blood vessels consist of a lengthy system of pipelines that measure on an average 60 thousands miles. These pipes are spread like roads and lanes and reach each and every cell in the body. The blood vessels are further classified into **arteries** and **veins**. Arteries carry blood away from the heart whereas veins bring blood back to the heart. The arteries are of following types

1. Large elastic arteries
2. Medium sized muscular arteries
3. Small arteries and smaller vessels called capillaries

The large arteries are like **highways**, medium arteries are like **roads** that run into organs and capillaries are like **lanes** that enter into every house or cell in the body. Veins finally **drain** the **arterial blood** that flows into the capillaries. The capillaries are very thin and form a network, a link between arteries and veins. These tiny capillaries pass through the tissue fluid and exchange of substances take place between tissue fluid and capillaries. For example, oxygen present in the blood within the capillaries passes out into the tissue fluid. It is picked up by the cells and the carbon dioxide, which is a waste, flows from the cells into tissue fluid from where it is carried away by the capillaries. In a similar manner, other substances like glucose are exchanged between cells and capillaries.

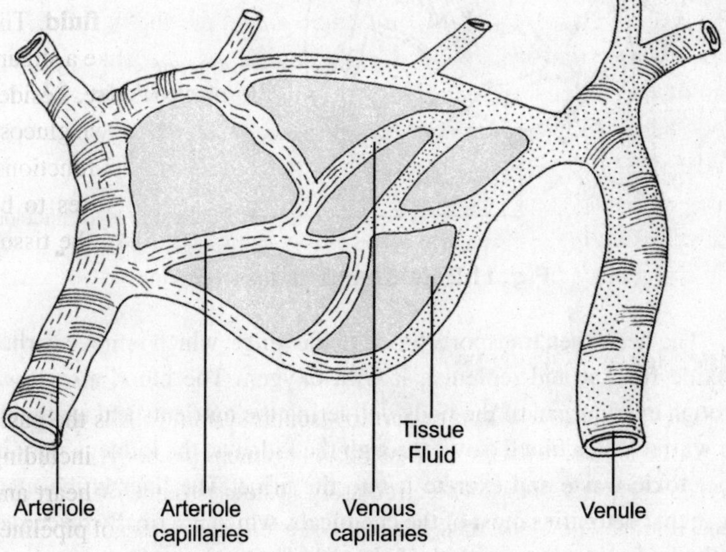

Fig. 11.1 Capillary Network

The Heart

The heart pumps the blood into the large blood vessels from where it is finally carried to the capillaries. It pumps blood hundred thousand times every day, hence, performing an enormous task. As the blood pools into the capillary meshwork, the nutrients and oxygen ooze out of the capillaries and pass into the tissue fluid from where these substances go into the cells. The waste is picked up by the capillaries from the tissue fluid, into which it has been excreted by the cells, and then taken back to the heart via the veins.

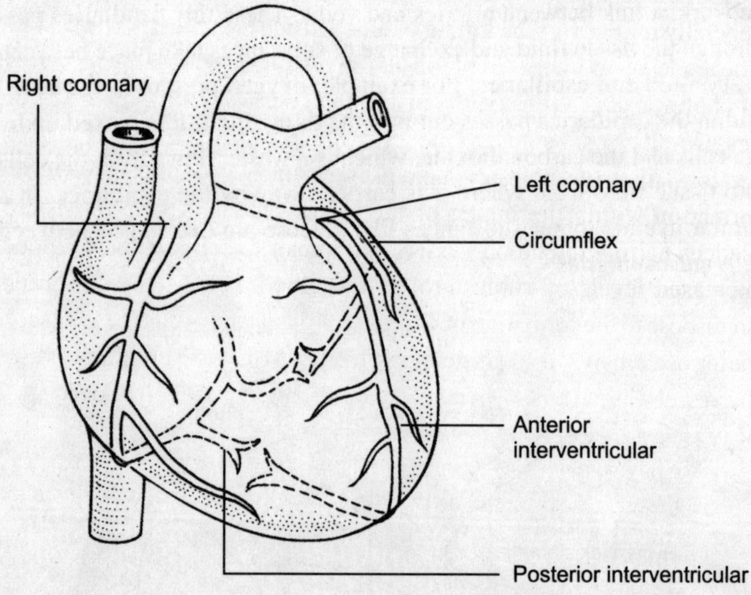

Fig. 11.2 Heart and its arteries

The heart then transports blood to the lungs, which remove carbon dioxide from it and replenish it with oxygen. The blood also flows through every organ of the body delivering the nutrients and removing the waste. When blood flows through the kidneys, the kidneys remove other toxic waste and excrete it into the urine. The liver is the main organ that detoxifies most of the chemicals, which are finally discarded by the body into urine with the help of kidneys.

A healthy body requires healthy cells. For healthy cells, it is vital that the cardiovascular system, which is the primary delivery network, should remain disease free and efficient. The pumping action of the heart and the pushing of the blood into the blood vessels occur by the alternate contraction and relaxation of the muscle cells present in the heart. The further flow of blood through the blood vessel network is achieved partly by the recoil of elastic vessels and partly by the contractile activity of muscular vessels.

Hypercholesteramia

Any clog in the pipeline of blood vessels may obstruct the free flow of blood and seriously impair the delivery system. These clogs are generally formed by the clotting of blood inside the lumen of the vessels. The tendency of increased blood clotting is subsequent to the formation of **cholesterol plaques** on the inside and consequent thickening of the vessel wall. Any damage to the inner lining of the wall predisposes to the formation of cholesterol plaques and increased tendency of clot formation within the lumen of the blood vessels. These cholesterol plaques narrow the blood vessels and impair the circulation of blood. Increased levels of cholesterol in the blood, due to any condition, predispose to the formation of cholesterol plaques and this in turn causes *arteriosclerosis. It also increases tendency of blood clotting within the vessel walls. Thus, hypercholesteramia, arteriosclerosis and clogging of vessels are closely interlinked.

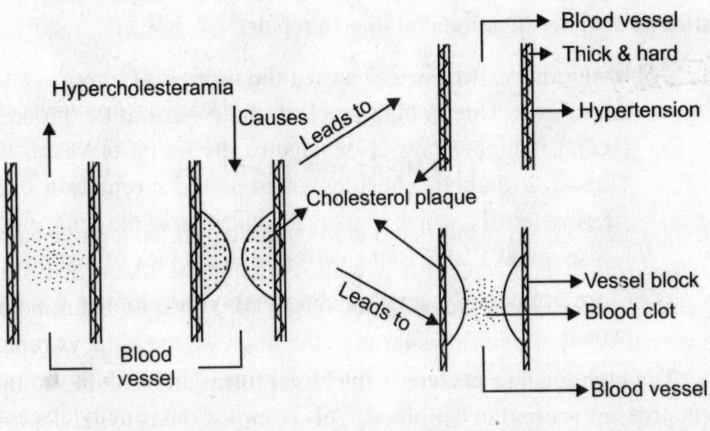

Fig. 11.3 Hypercholesteramia, Cholesterol Plaques, Hypertension and Clot formation and Vessel Block.

Any damage to the muscle cells of the heart may also adversely affect the efficiency of the cardiovascular activity. A diabetic is more prone to arteriosclerosis, as the cholesterol levels are high in these persons. As a result, the circulation in these patients is often compromised. The vessels which supply blood to the muscles of the heart called **coronary vessels**, may also get affected and in such situations the cells of the heart suffer damage.

A natural wear and tear goes on in the body. The body is endowed with the ability to heal and repair This ability to repair is, however, limited only to some tissues in the body. Some cells like neurons in the brain and spinal cord, muscle cells of the heart, once damaged, do not repair and regenerate. Similarly pancreatic islet cells, if damaged, are lost forever as they lack the biological ability to repair.

However, the skin cells and the cells lining the cavities of hollow organs and tube like structures such as the blood vessels, have tremendous power to multiply and replenish the lost cell mass. If the cells of the blood vessel are damaged at a higher rate, which frequently happens in diabetes, the process of arteriosclerosis is hastened. Vitamins and especially vitamin C, is an important ingredients necessary for the healing mechanism.

In a diabetic, the blood glucose levels are high. The cells are starved, as glucose is unable to enter the cells either due to lack of insulin or insensitivity of the cells to insulin. As a result, the nutrition of the cells suffer as also the functional ability to repair.

- In summary, two factors hasten the process of arteriosclerosis in diabetes. One is high level of cholesterol in the blood and second is higher rate of damage to the lining of vessel wall. Thus in a diabetic, besides an impaired circulation due to arteriosclerosis, which impairs the nutrition of the cells, glucose is also not available to the cells due to the lack of insulin.
- More importantly, another abnormality develops in a diabetic patient.

The high glucose present in the blood forms an insoluble complex with proteins present in the blood. This complex tends to get deposited on the wall of the small blood vessels and occlude them. This seriously impairs circulation, especially the microcirculation and further compromises nutrition of the cells of the body.

Advanced Glycosylation End Products (AGE) are formed when blood glucose binds with different proteins in the blood. These form insoluble compounds that tend to deposit on the blood vessel wall, thereby narrowing the lumen of the blood vessels.

In response to the lack of utilization of glucose, the fats are mobilized from the adipose tissue, into the blood and taken to the liver for further metabolism. The liver subsequently metabolizes the fats and throws them back into the circulating blood. The resulting high levels of LDL in the blood are very harmful as these are closely linked to atherosclerosis/arteriosclerosis.

Atherosclerosis

Atherosclerosis is a disease of large and medium sized blood vessels. This is an ageing process of blood vessels that not only affects the elderly but also the young. In this condition, plaques develop on the walls of blood vessels, which narrow and constrict them. These plaques are made up of **cholesterol**. The cholesterol comes from the blood stream into the plaques. **LDL cholesterol** is the one, which forms the **plaques**. But before entry into the vessel wall, LDL in the blood is first oxidized and then picked up by the macrophages (the scavenger cells of the body), which exist in the walls of blood vessels, thereby getting LDL deposited in the plaques.

Why LDL is so closely associated with atherosclerosis is not exactly known. When the level of LDL in the blood is high that of HDL is low in almost in an inverse ratio. HDL is a protective fat and helps to lower the risk of arteriosclerosis. The level of LDL cholesterol is high in diabetics, making them more prone to atherosclerosis. The pre-request for the deposition of LDL in the vessel wall is its oxidation. The anti-oxidants present in our meals help to hinder the oxidation and help to reduce the formation of **atherosclerotic plaques**.

Arteriosclerosis

Arteriosclerosis is a disease, which affects many blood vessels but chiefly the **coronary** and **carotid vessels** bear the brunt. The coronary vessels nourish the heart muscles. When circulation in the coronary arteries is compromised, oxygen supply to the muscle cells decrease and patient feels pain or sense of constriction in the chest. These are some of the symptoms of **angina**. If the blood and oxygen supply to the heart is completely blocked, when a vessel is occluded by a blood clot, a portion of the heart, which is deprived of oxygen, undergoes degeneration or death resulting in heart attack. A similar situation can occur in carotid arteries, which are blood vessels carrying blood to the brain and lead to stroke.

In obese persons, the fat cells present inside the abdominal cavity produce a substance called **plasminogen-activator inhibitor**. This substance prevents dissolution of blood clots within the blood vessels and thereby predisposes to **heart attack** and **stroke**. Therefore, obese persons are at greater risk to coronary heart disease and stroke.

When the blood supply to the kidneys is compromised, degenerative changes take place in the kidneys. Also, kidney starts producing a substance called **angiotensin**, which raises the **blood pressure**. High blood pressure or hypertension is a common complication of diabetes. Hypertension further aggravates arteriosclerosis.

There is also dysfunction of the lining cells of the blood vessels in diabetes. These cells are called the **endothelial cells**. As a result of dysfunction of these cells, the proper dilatation of the blood vessels also suffers.

Various Physiological Malfunctioning in Diabetes

1. **The impaired circulation** in diabetes affects the nutrition of each and every cell in the body and compromises the efficient functioning of every organ and system in the body. As the nutrition of the nervous system suffers, various types of **neurological symptoms** as numbness, tingling, burning, loss of sensations in hands and feet, and sciatica type of pain occurs. In a diabetic patient, the circulation of the blood in the blood vessels gets compromised due to following three factors.

   (i) The increased incidence of arteriosclerosis in diabetes.

   (ii) The increased deposition of protein-glucose complex inside the vessel walls.

(iii) The endothelial cell dysfunction resulting in the decreased vasodilatation.

2. The patient often misses a small cut in the feet due to the loss of sensations in the feet. Due to the **poor vitality** of **skin** and underlying tissues, the wound refuse to heal, leading to a **non-healing wound**. The infection in the wound may also advance so far as to necessitate amputation. As the immune system is also at low ebb, serious infections can occur and patient takes longer time to overcome any infection.
3. In diabetes, the patient presents symptoms of excessive thirst, hunger and urination. His blood sugar level is very high and often above 180 mg%. Whenever blood sugar level exceeds 180 mg%, sugar spills into urine. This raises the osmolarity of urine and the kidney tubules suck out water from the blood to balance the **osmotic pressure**. More urine is formed resulting in increased urination. This in turn leads to dehydration and the patient feels thirsty.
4. Due to the inability to utilize glucose, the patient also feels very hungry. The brain depends largely on glucose for its energy needs and when glucose is not available either because it is low or insulin is low; the person feels dizzy and even faints. Due to the lack of glucose utilization, fats are mobilized into the circulation in the form of ketone bodies. Excessive accumulation of ketone bodies in circulation causes ketosis, which is a life threatening condition.

Due to the lack of utilization of glucose, the body fat is broken down to meet the energy demands of the body resulting in loss of weight. Along with fat, the body also breaks down muscle proteins. As a result, the person becomes lean and thin.

Somogyi Effect

This effect is a **rebound phenomenon** in which the body reacts to extremely **low blood sugar levels** by overcompensating, resulting in high sugar levels. When blood glucose falls, which sometimes happens in the middle of the night, the body secretes counter regulatory hormones such as glucagons** and epinephrine***.

These hormones make the liver convert glycogen (present in its stores) into glucose; pour it into the blood, thereby raising the blood glucose levels. This happens when the night dose of insulin is more or the food intake at dinner is less. The **Somogyi effect** can be avoided by preventing **hypoglycemia** in the first place. This requires proper insulin dose and proper meal planning at dinner.

---

* Glucagon is a hormone, secreted by the alpha cells present in the islets of Langerhans in the pancreas. The action of this hormone is opposite to that of insulin.

** Epinephrine or adrenaline is secreted by adrenal glands, which are situated close to the kidneys. This hormone also raises blood sugar levels.

*** Arteriosclerosis means thickening and hardening of the vessel, often resulting in hypertension.

Chapter 12

COMPLICATIONS OF DIABETES

The morbidity and mortality of complications of diabetes is so profound that no message is strong enough to beat the menace. The more you know about it the less it is. A brief outline of various complications, such as lipid disorders, hypertension, heart attack, stroke, blindness, kidney failure and numerous neuropathies is given in this chapter. Dental complications, non-healing wounds, impaired immunity and skin disorders are also discussed. Serious problems that need immediate hospitalization are also mentioned.

Serious complications can occur in diabetes including heart attack, hypertension, blindness, life threatening infections, kidney failure, non-healing wounds and amputation. The benefits of rigid control of diabetes lasts for years, according to the recent follow up study by DCCT (Diabetes Control and Complication Trial) of NIH. The tight control of diabetes and continuing medical assessment of the patient also delays the onset of eye and kidney complications. Researchers from the **United Kingdom Prospective Diabetic Study** (UKPDS) group have also given substantial evidence that strict glycemic control can delay or prevent the onset of complications of diabetes.

Prevention of these complications remain an important element in the total management of diabetes. Recognition of the various precipitating factors that induce complications and correct knowledge of the appropriate instructions that need to be carried out will go a long way in decreasing the incidence of these complications. **Self-care, awareness** and **vigilance** in such situations help to **reduce morbidity** and **mortality** in this disease.

Lipid Disorders

All diabetics, young and old, must get their lipid profile evaluated at the time of diagnosis and later at regular intervals. In adults with diabetes mellitus, the LDL cholesterol should be < 100 mg/dl, HDL cholesterol > 45 mg/dl and triglycerides < 200 mg/dl. Certain thyroid disorders, such as hypothyroidism, can also elevate lipid levels. These may coexist with diabetes and should be ruled out. In case there is thyroid hormone deficiency, it should be corrected.

The Scandinavian Simvastatin Survival study demonstrated that the use of **simvastatin**, a **cholesterol lowering drug,** resulted in an average of 35% decrease of LDL cholesterol and the reduction of coronary mortality by 42%. Co-existing conditions and disorders, such as smoking, hypertension, premature CHD (coronary heart disease) and familial hypercholesteremia should be taken into consideration while targeting lipid levels. Statins are generally well tolerated and consequently these are chosen as the first line of action in treating diabetic dyslipidemia. When the levels of triglycerides are high, fibric acid derivatives, another class of lipid lowering drugs may be considered after obtaining optimal glycemic control. When using combination therapy, it is recommended that low doses of statins be used, as then they have been found to be safer.

Coronary Heart Disease and Hypertension

Patients with diabetes are at higher risk of developing high blood pressure also called **hypertension**. It is estimated that about 60 - 65% of patients with diabetes develop hypertension. Hypertension further raises the risk of heart disease, which is already high in diabetics. It also increases the risk of **diabetic retinopathy**. UKPDS trials showed that hypertension was associated with the increased risk of all complications. The tight control of blood pressure decreased the overall risk by nearly 24% in all end stage conditions linked with the diabetes. Hypertension further accelerates arteriosclerosis and decreases blood supply to the tissues. So, it is very important to have a rigid control of blood pressure. UKPDS group also revealed that blood pressure control decreased the risk of stroke in patients of type 2diabetes. It demonstrated that improved blood pressure control resulted in a 44% reduction in the risk of fatal and nonfatal strokes.

American Diabetes Association recommends that all patients with diabetes should have their blood pressure less than 130 mm/Hg systolic and 85 mm/Hg diastolic. The National Center for **Chronic Disease Prevention and Health Promotion, Centers for Disease Control and Prevention, Atlanta,** Georgia, has shown that US control of hypertension is not adequate. The investigators concluded that 71% adult diabetics had high blood pressure and the incidence increased with age and was elevated in both sexes as well as in non-Hispanic blacks and non-Hispanic whites. Of all the persons with elevated blood pressure, only 71% were aware of their condition and only 57% were taking the treatment. Control of blood pressure was least common among elderly patients. Just as it is important to **control blood sugar**, it is equally important to **control blood pressure**. Patients, whose blood pressure was controlled, had reduced risk of heart attack, stroke and angina. A **regular check up of blood pressure is essential**. Smoking and alcohol tend to raise the blood pressure especially in already predisposed persons like diabetics. Mild hypertension can be controlled by few simple measures. These include control of body weight, reduction in the intake of alcohol, decrease in salt intake, and reduction in smoking. In case these measures fail or the hypertension is marked then medical consultation and medication is required.

Antihypertensive Drugs

Among the **antihypertensive agents** used are ACE (angiotensin converting enzyme) inhibitors. They have been found to be effective and well tolerated and have favourable effects in reducing microalbuminuria (discussed later in text) and nephropathy. The ACE inhibitors have no adverse effect on glucose or insulin levels and some studies have shown improved insulin sensitivity. There use is contraindicated in pregnant women. Other anti-hypertensive drugs as beta-blockers and calcium channel blockers are also effective. Salt restriction and low fat diet is strongly recommended.

High levels of LDL cholesterol and triglycerides contribute to this process of arteriosclerosis. Several studies have revealed that lipid-lowering drugs reduce the incidence of coronary artery disease. The **Scandinavian Simvastatin Survival Study** demonstrated that simvastatin resulted in an average reduction of LDL by 35%, reducing coronary mortality by 42% and total mortality by 30%. Their data also showed that treating patients of diabetes with simvastatin lowered the incidence of coronary events in hyperlipidemic cases by 55%. **Cholesterol and Recurrent Events (CARE)** Study revealed that **pravastatin**, another cholesterol-lowering drug, was effective in reducing the risk of CAD by 25% in patients with diabetes and 23% in patients without diabetes. One tablet of aspirin or micropyrin of 75-150 mgs taken daily, helps to prevent clotting of blood and goes a long way in the prevention of heart attacks. This is to be taken under medical considerations.

In diabetics as compared to non-diabetic subjects, heart disease appears earlier in life in the diabetics. Also, it affects men and women alike and is more often fatal.

Deaths due to heart attack are 20% more in diabetics as compared to the non-diabetic patients. About 70-80% of diabetic adults die of coronary artery disease, stroke or peripheral vascular disease. This incidence is 2-4 times more as compared to non-diabetic adults.

Rigid and strict control of blood glucose levels and blood pressure significantly reduces the risk of these complications. The incidence of repeat heart attack is also more in diabetics as compared to non-diabetics. The most common cause of death in adults with diabetes is **coronary heart disease**. About 9% of diabetic adults suffer from stroke. The thickening and narrowing of the vessels, which take place in the coronary blood vessels, also take place in the blood vessels of the brain.

Heart attacks and strokes occur due to the decrease of blood supply to these vital organs. The decrease of blood supply is due to the thickening and rigidity of the wall of blood vessels as well as the narrowing of their lumen. This is the result of fats getting deposited on the wall of the blood vessels. If blood clots within these narrowed vessels the result is complete blockage of the vessels.

Lower Extremity Arterial Disease (LEAD)

Lower extremity arterial disease (LEAD) is identified by the absence or deficit in peripheral pulses in lower legs and feet. It represents decreased blood supply and reduced arterial perfusion of extremities. It causes **intermittent claudication**. The patient experiences pain while walking and it disappear on resting. In population-based studies, pulse deficits were found in 10% of diabetic adults, absent pulse in 20-30% of cases and about 9% of diabetics suffered from intermittent claudication. The incidence increases with older age, longer duration of diabetes, cigarette smoking, hypertension and dyslipidaemia.

LEAD further aggravates the situation when compounded with peripheral neuropathy and increased susceptibility to infection.

Insulin Resistance Syndrome

Insulin Resistance Syndrome (IRS) is also known as syndrome **X/ CHOAS**. It stands for **Coronary artery disease, hypertension, obesity, atherosclerosis** and **stroke**. The exact genesis of insulin resistance has not been elucidated. One theory pronounces that high levels of fatty acids in blood circulation of obese individuals block insulin receptors on tissue cells and cause insulin resistance.

IRS could have a genetic basis. It is a vicious cycle. High levels of insulin in the blood cause obesity, as insulin favors lipogenesis, and obesity in turn produces insulin resistance and high insulin production by the pancreas.

This syndrome is associated with the obese type 2diabetes mellitus and it sometimes presents in persons even before the disease is recognized and the diagnosis is established. Such individuals, besides being obese, are characterized by high levels of insulin in blood. This is also seen in persons with **impaired glucose tolerance (IGT)**. Besides diabetes, this syndrome is also associated with hyperlipidemia, hyperinsulinemia, hypertension, coronary heart disease and stroke.

IRS is seen in many US adults. Smoking, lack of exercise and high carbohydrate consumption predispose to IRS. Control of body weight and change of sedentary life style, lesser intake of fats and cholesterol, adequate control of diabetes help in decreasing insulin resistance and alleviating the risk of complications.

Another theory proposes that **PC-1 protein** interfere with the normal functioning of **insulin receptors**. The level of this protein is higher in type 2diabetes as compared to normal persons. The synthesis of this protein is genetically determined.

Scientists have suggested that intake of low fat dairy products and calcium may discourage the development of IRS.

Diabetic Eye Disease

Eye and vision disturbances are very common in diabetics. A regular eye check-up is mandatory in diabetics. In a diabetic, following symptoms should be taken seriously and visual disturbances call for immediate medical considerations.

- Loss of peripheral vision,
- Hazy vision,
- Presence of floaters,
- Flashes or any visual disturbance.

One day, a friend of mine came to me and complained that his vision had become hazy. When I tested his blood sugar, it was found to be elevated, more than 300 mgs%. He had been careless with his control of diet and diabetes. The hazy vision frightened him. He went on strict dietary regime and a more rigid control of his diabetes, regularly monitoring his blood sugar levels. The visual defect, as told by the ophthalmologist was due to early cataract. Strict control of diabetes hindered further progression of the disease.

According to a study published in a medical journal, high levels of an amino acid called homocysteine may increase the risk of damage to the eye and its nerves causing blindness. In a research carried out in Netherlands patients of diabetes having high levels of homocysteine in blood, were at higher risk of developing eye damage and blindness. In uncontrolled diabetes, a number of following eye problems can occur.

1. Diabetic Retinopathy
2. Cataract
3. Glaucoma

Diabetic Retinopathy

It is the leading cause of blindness among **American adults**. Between 12,000 and 24,000 new cases of blindness due to diabetic retinopathy occur each year. It is twice as common as cataract and glaucoma among persons with diabetes. The prevalence of this complication is strongly related to the duration of the illness. Nearly all cases of type 1diabetes, develop retinopathy after 20 years duration, as also more than 60% of type 2diabetes. Research has revealed that poor control of diabetes has strong association with retinopathy. Strict control of blood glucose levels not only prevents but also delays the development and slows the progression of this complication.

The blood vessels of the retina, which is the innermost coat of the eyeball, having the photoreceptors that visualize light, are affected. They undergo distortion, becoming narrow at some points and widened at others. As a result, the permeability of the vessels is affected causing abnormal exudation of plasma and hemorrhages into the retina. As a result of exudation into the macular area, there is **macular edema**. Macula, an area in the retina, which is also called the yellow spot has maximum visual acuity. Hence, edema in the macular area adversely affects eyesight. The **edema** and **hemorrhages** into the retina may seriously impair the visual acuity and may lead to blindness. There is no pain and the symptoms may not appear before the disease is fairly well advanced. The longer a person suffers from diabetes the more the chances of **developing retinopathy**.

Early detection of this condition can help reduce the morbidity, as laser treatment is very effective in this condition. Hence, it is imperative that every patient must have his eyes examined regularly, at least once a year, after getting the pupils dilated so as to permit the complete viewing of the inner chamber of the eye. **Laser treatment** has decreased the incidence of severe visual impairment by nearly 60%.

- I remember another patient, Ms D, a music teacher, pretty and petite, with life full of dreams and expectations. Then suddenly disaster struck. Even as she played the piano, one day, she could not read the book as her vision blurred. She panicked and consulted the doctor and was found to be diabetic. She had developed retinopathy. Treatment prevented total blindness.
- I recall another case. Our teacher and professor of surgery, in a leading medical institute, lost his eyesight due to retinal detachment. After this episode and after much motivation, he began to live life anew. Though the outside world had become dark, he rekindled a lamp in his heart. With proper medication and a strict, disciplined life, he lived healthily for many years and even took active part in social functions. As the saying goes every cloud has a silver lining.

Cataract

Cataract means clouding or **opacification of lens** of the eye. The high blood glucose levels lead to the tendency of glucose oozing out into the lens substance, wherein it forms a complex with lens proteins. This is an insoluble compound and precipitates into the lens substance. Cataract as a rule develops in old age as a part of **ageing process**. In diabetics, there is early and premature development of cataract.

Glaucoma

Glaucoma indicates an increase in the pressure of fluid within the eyeball. This increased pressure presses on the retina and optic nerve and leads to optic nerve atrophy* and impairment of vision. This occurs due to the proliferation of blood vessels in the iris and the ciliary body, leading to increased oozing out of tissue fluid from these capillary channels, and its accumulation in the chamber of eyeball.

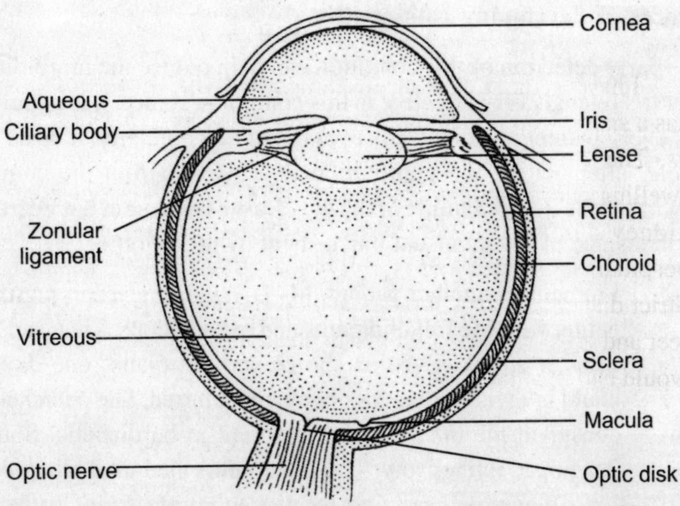

Fig. 12.1 Horizontal section of the eyeball.

Kidney Disease

The ADA (American Diabetes Association) has reported that in the USA, more than 20,000 patients with diabetes are diagnosed with

End Stage Renal Disease (ESRD) every year. Diabetes is the most common cause of end stage renal disease. It is more common in African-Americans and Native-Americans for reasons unknown. As shown by the DCCT and UKPDS trials, intensive control of blood glucose in patients significantly reduces the risk of kidney damage and prevents or delays end stage renal disease.

Symptoms of kidney disease or nephropathy usually occur in the late stages of the disease, when kidney functions have fallen to 25% of the normal. The earliest clinical sign of nephropathy is **microalbuminuria**, which means the loss of albumin in urine exceeding 30 mg/day. The loss of albumin > 300 mg/day is present in frank nephropathy. ESRD develops in 50% of type 1diabetes in 10 years time, and in 75% by 20 years. About 20-40% of type 2diabetes also progress to overt nephropathy, if specific intervention is not provided. In 20% cases of type 2diabetes, ESRD develops by 20 years.

Case Story 1

I have a friend, who is a diabetic and visits us quite often. She has a sister, who is also diabetic and one day both of them came to us. The sister was not feeling well and complained of massive swelling over both feet and lower legs. I knew she had developed kidney dysfunction and needed specialist care and possibly hospitalization for few days. Her blood sugar levels were very high. Strict diabetic control and medication reduced the swelling on her feet and legs. She was told that if she continues to be careless she would end in renal failure.

Case Story 2

Here is a patient whom I pity. Rich and famous, he had scant respect for diet control and discipline, despite being obese and diabetic. Words of caution would be drowned in a resounding guffaw and he continued with his indulgence in fatty food and sweets. Soon, diabetes struck him where it hurt and it proved fatal. He developed diabetic nephropathy and died of kidney failure. Diabetes is a wild animal unless tamed.

Kidney Function Tests

The blood supply to the kidney gets compromised over a period of time due to the narrowing of blood vessels. This change occurs more often in type 1diabetes as compared to type 2. Also, the changes are more marked and appear earlier in type 1diabetes. Kidney function tests should be carried out from time to time after nephropathy has been detected. When nephropathy develops:

- Low protein diet is advocated.
- A strict glycemic control is mandatory.
- If hypertension coexists, it should be treated seriously and adequately.
- Lipid levels should be rigidly controlled.

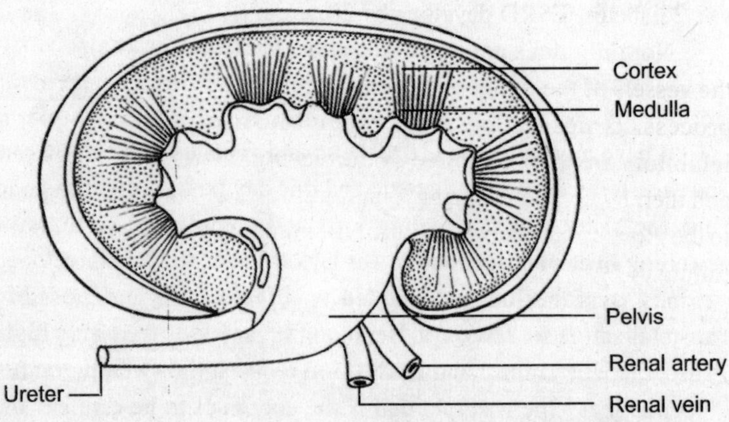

Fig. 12.2 Cross-section of human kidney

Structure of Kidney

The functional unit of the kidney is called **nephron**, which is made up of **glomerulus** and the **tubules**. The glomerulus consists of a meshwork of tiny blood vessels, which filters the blood brought to the kidney by larger blood vessels and removes body waste that flows down the renal tubules. By virtue of its filtration process and differential absorption in the tubules, not only the toxic waste is removed from the body but also the salt-water balance and acid-base equilibrium of body is preserved. As the vessels of the glomerulus get thickened and narrowed over a period of time, the filtration process gets continuously impaired. The earliest manifestation of glomerular damage is the presence of tiny traces of albumin in the urine.

Albumin is a **protein present in the blood**. With the impairment of glomerular function, albumin begins to leak into the urine. This is called **microalbuminuria**. It is the earliest clinical sign of nephropathy (kidney disease). Loss of more than 30 mg/day of albumin is considered microalbuminuria. As damage increases more albumin is lost into the urine. The loss of protein in the urine may be very massive or very minute. The loss of protein from the body leads to other metabolic abnormalities. The degenerative changes in the kidney lead to the ultimate production of angiotensin by the tubules of the kidney. Angiotensin is the substance, which causes hypertension.

Not only does angiotensin cause hypertension, it also narrows the vessels of the glomerulus and further aggravates the degenerative process. Drugs called **ACE (angiotensin converting enzyme)** inhibitors are very effective in decreasing the levels of angiotensin and thereby help in lowering hypertension and decreasing the damage to the glomerulus. Degeneration of the kidney ultimately ends in kidney failure.

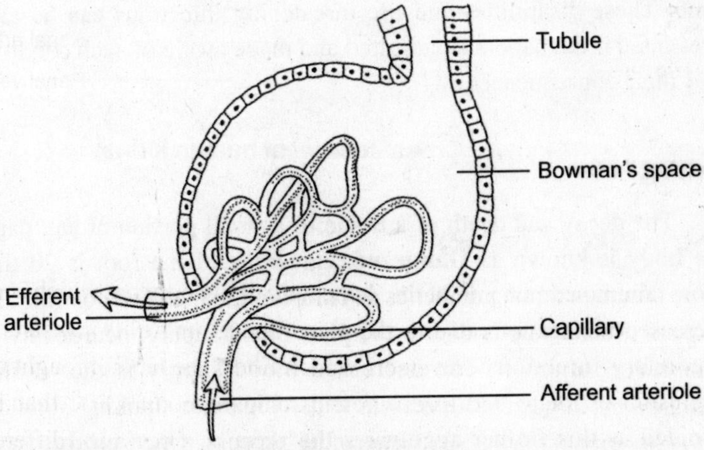

Fig. 12.3 Glomerulus

Non-Healing Wounds

In diabetics, the wounds take a long time to heal. This is because of the poor vitality and reduced healing power of the tissues due to decreased blood supply, as well as the immune system being at low ebb.

I know of a young boy, eight years old suffering from type 1diabetes. He is always reluctant to play with his classmates on the playground, for whenever he falls and gets a cut or scratch on the body, the wound takes a long time to heal.

Non-healing wounds can occur anywhere in the body, but occur more commonly on those parts of the body that are under pressure. Persons with impaired mobility, such as those who are bedridden or those who are confined to wheelchair or even those who are obese, have a greater tendency to **develop ulcers**. Such ulcers develop on pressure points like the buttocks and feet especially undersurface of great toe and heel, as the blood supply to these areas gets restricted due to pressure, more so in an already compromised situation as occurs in a diabetic. If the wound does not hurt it is worst still, as that indicates loss of sensation, one of the features of neuropathy. Due to the loss of sensation a small scratch or cut often goes unnoticed and neglected. This can lead to inadequate treatment of the wound that may ultimately result in serious infection and a nonhealing wound. More than 60% of diabetic ulcers get infected and many require amputation of foot or limb. These disabilities and life threatening infections can be easily prevented if the patient is educated and made aware of such conditions and their consequences.

Gangrene

The decay and death of a tissue or a small portion of any part of the body is known as **Gangrene**. Gangrene of the foot is 20 times more common among diabetics as compared to matched controls. This increased incidence is due to the poor blood supply, neuropathy and secondary infection. The decreased blood supply is the result of occlusion of micro and macro vessels. Cigarette smoking should be avoided as this further aggravates the process. Once ulceration and gangrene sets in, the treatment is **extremely difficult**.

Case Story 3

Here I am reminded of another incident. He was a good friend of ours and had diabetes. Always smiling and bubbly, he took life in a lighter vein as also his diabetes, till a minor scratch took away his foot. It was an injury, just a scratch that refused to heal. It got infected and gangrene developed. Despite best efforts and treatment, his leg had to be amputated as the deadly gangrene spread upwards and consumed the limb. It was tragic fallout of uncontrolled diabetes.

Diabetic Neuropathy

Diabetic neuropathy is a disorder that affects the nervous system of the body and about 60% patients show some kind of nerve damage. This is more common in patients with uncontrolled diabetes, and in whom the blood glucose level has remained elevated for 10 years or more. It can affect both types of diabetes. Alcohol and smoking also increase the risk of developing diabetic neuropathy and they can worsen the existing state of the condition. Strict glucose control may delay the progression or prevent the development of neuropathy.

Diabetic neuropathy can involve the sensory, the motor and the autonomic nerves. The sensory and motor nerves belong to the voluntary nervous system and the autonomic nerves belong to the involuntary nervous system. The voluntary nervous system supplies the skeletal muscles and skin and is under the conscious control of the mind. The involuntary nervous system innervates the internal organs and is beyond the conscious control of the mind. The **microangiopathy** that occurs in DM, results in decreased blood supply to the nerves, and damage to the nerves. The damage to the nerves may also result from metabolic affects of diabetes. Some of these changes are reversible in the early stages, if the diabetes is brought under control.

Sensory Disturbances

Sensory disturbances pertain to sensations of the body. There may be loss or decreased sensations or feeling of abnormal sensations. These disturbances may be of following types.

1. In **distal polyneuropathy**, the distal portions of the limbs, which mean the hands, feet and the adjoining portion of the arms and

legs, are affected in glove and stocking pattern. Distal means the **involvement of the peripheral nerves**, and polyneuropathy means **multiple nerve involvement**. The sensory system is the first to be affected and perception of pain, touch and temperature becomes dull. The patient may feel abnormal sensations such as tingling, burning, crawling of ants, or extreme cold in hands or feet. The patient may feel as if he is walking on rocks or may not feel the firmness of ground beneath the feet.

2. There may be loss of balance and coordination.
3. Insensitivity to pain may be so much that small cuts in the feet go unfelt and therefore unnoticed.
4. Sometimes, the involvement of the roots of the nerves results in excruciating pain in the area of distribution of the nerve supply, for example resembling sciatica.

All these symptoms are worse at night

Case Study 4

Another case comes to my mind. Mrs. Sangeeta, aged 46, was of nervous temperament. She often felt a burning and pricking sensation on the soles of her feet, as if walking on rocks. Her friends and relatives felt she was crazy. She kept visiting a psychiatrist but though she found some mental solace, her disease was not healed, as it did not exactly lie in the mind. Later she went to a doctor who tested her for diabetes. She tested positive and was treated for diabetes. She recovered from the affliction and the lost self-esteem.

Case Story 5

This takes me back several years, when such a case occurred. It was a mid-life affliction when life was in full sail and there was not much to worry for tomorrow. Active, athletic and in his forties, Mr. Sethi never forget to take time off for a few minutes of exercise. A shooting pain in his lower back pinned him down, even as he was stretching his legs during his morning workout. He thought he had pulled a muscle. Recurring pain troubled him and he began popping in painkillers. But his discomfort continued. His youthful spirit was caged and wrinkles grew on his face. He finally came to us and blood sugar estimation established the diagnosis of diabetes. A rigid control of diabetes alleviated his symptoms.

Motor Disturbances

1. The damage to motor nerves, which innervate the muscles of the hand and feet, may cause weakness of the movements of hands and feet.
2. Involvement of some nerves can cause weakness of the muscles that move the eyeball, resulting in diplopia or double vision.
3. If the nerve supplying the muscles of the face is affected, then eye-lid may droop or the mouth may not close fully and food may dribble out.

Case Story 6

An elderly gentleman, a known diabetic, started seeing double. He became upset and anxious. He tested his blood sugar and found it to be extremely high. He realized he had been careless with his diabetic control. That was an eye-opener. He consulted an ophthalmologist who told him that focal nerve palsy of muscle of the eyeball had caused it. The condition was self-limiting and symptoms regressed in few weeks.

Focal neuropathy occurs most frequently in older patients. Specific nerves are affected, more often in the torso, head and leg. The onset of symptoms is sudden and self-limiting.

It can cause problems of hearing and even facial paralysis, difficulty in focusing, and double vision, when nerves of the head are involved. Severe pain in the lower back or pelvis, in the chest, stomach and thigh may occur. Pain in the chest may mimic heart attack.

Autonomic Disturbances

Autonomic neuropathy affects the nerves supplying the internal organs of the body. The damage to the autonomic nerves may cause the following.

1. Gastrointestinal disturbances such as bouts of diarrhoea and constipation. When the nerves of the stomach are involved, the stomach fails to empty in normal time and food does not enter

the intestine and hence fails to get digested on time. This results in brittle diabetes as the blood glucose levels fluctuate wildly, as while the anti-diabetic drugs continue to be active, glucose fails to reach the blood stream due to delay in its absorption. Diarrhoea may be very severe and there may be more than ten motions in a day.

2. The nerve damage to the muscles of the urinary bladder may result in inability to empty the urinary bladder completely. Due to the loss of sensation of bladder fullness and inability to contract the bladder muscles, there is loss of bladder control and loss of its adequate and complete emptying. This results in the stagnation of urine inside the bladder, which in turn predisposes to urinary tract infection.
3. Impotence in both man and woman. Man may have difficulty in attaining and maintaining an erection. Woman may experience inability to achieve orgasm.
4. Postural hypotension, which means sudden fall in blood pressure on standing up from lying down posture, can also occur.
5. Lack of sweating may occur in the feet.
6. In the late stages, the heart may fail to speed up with exercise. Patient may not feel chest pain during heart attacks, and thus have an attack without being aware of it.
7. Bile may stagnate in gall bladder due to failure of contraction of the muscles of the bile passage and predispose to the formation of gallstones.
8. Patients may have difficulty in sensing hypoglycemia.

Many drugs are available for the treatment of neurological complications. These include anti-depressants, anti-epileptics and painkillers. Acupuncture has also been tried as also electrical stimulation of painful nerve endings.

Sexual Dysfunction

Sex and love intricately weave into man's happiness. Unsatisfactory sex life leaves man distraught and miserable. Diabetics may face a number of sex inadequacies and disturbances. But these are not such, that cannot be handled or treated. Such individuals should not feel shy or hesitate in discussing their problems with their doctors. They should not deny themselves the basic instinct and pleasure.

Man often experience lack of erection. This could be the result of vascular, neurological or psychological reasons. Impotence may be failure to have or sustain erection. Man feels fewer, less firm erection, and those that do not last long enough. This, in turn fails to arouse orgasm in the sex partner. Impotence often increases with age and with duration of diabetes. Excessive intake of alcoholic drinks, smoking and intake of drugs such as opiates also aggravate it.

Woman often feels lack of sexual desire. Beside diminished sexual response during intercourse, woman may experience vaginal pain that may get aggravated by fungal infection in the vagina. A diabetic woman is quite prone to **fungal vaginitis.** There is also the problem of increased vaginal dryness. This could be due to the decrease in sex hormones in advancing age and diabetic process. Intercourse can produce hypoglycemia, especially in man. It is good to have a candy at hand. All these conditions can be easily treated by medicines. However, good blood sugar control underlines all therapies.

Case Story 7

Here is an incidence of pre-marital blues. An associate, he was the most eligible bachelor. A young man in his early thirties, was handsome and of royal lineage. He had the trappings of power, wealth and luxury, but he refused to marry. Being the only son, there was immense pressure from his parents to tie the knot and carry forward the lineage. But he kept spurning offers. He confided in another friend that he had difficulty in having erections. He made several rounds of quacks, who offered aphrodisiacs at a premium. One day, he confided in me and I advised him to take some tests including blood sugar estimation. He turned out to be diabetic. After medication and control of his diabetes, he got reprieve from impotence.

Impaired Immunity

Due to depressed immune response, diabetics are more susceptible to infections. Studies indicate that:

- There is higher risk of surgical wound infection, as in hip replacement operation.
- Greater chance of reactivation of tuberculosis and beta streptococcal infections.
- There is higher mortality from influenza and pneumonia.
- The incidence of urinary tract infection in women with diabetes is higher compared to non-diabetic adults.

Skin Diseases

There are several diseases of the skin to which a diabetic patient becomes predisposed. These conditions are listed below:

1. Patient is susceptible to both bacterial and fungal infections. A small cut or abrasion, if infected, can develop into a boil or carbuncle and then it requires aggressive therapy. Fungal infection can develop in between the toes, especially if the feet remain warm and moist.
2. Alopecia or loss of hair can develop in type 1diabetes.
3. Vitiligo or loss of normal skin pigmentation may develop in type 1diabetes.
4. Diabetics can develop thick dry skin.
5. Insulin hypertrophy or accumulation of fat at the site of insulin injections can occur.
6. Insulin lipoatrophy or loss of fat at the site of insulin injections can occur.

Dental Complications

Poor blood glucose control can result in **gingivitis, tooth decay** and **periodontal** disease. The thickening of blood vessels in a diabetic patient reduces the blood supply to the gums, thereby reducing the supply of oxygen and vital nutrients to the gums. This decreases the resistance of the gums to infections. Moreover, the high levels of glucose in the environment allow the bacteria in the mouth to thrive. So when diabetes is poorly controlled, the high glucose levels in the mouth added to poor resistance of the gums help bacteria to proliferate and cause gingivitis, where the gums become swollen, red and painful. If untreated and allowed to continue, this will progress into **periodontitis**. It is the infection and inflammation of the tissues around the teeth. The pocket of infection around the teeth may burrow deeper to infect the bony socket holding the teeth. The affected teeth may loosen and fall off. Hence to avoid dental complications, it is wise to control diabetes. To maintain good dental health of teeth :

- Avoid starchy food that stick to teeth,
- Regularly brush your teeth with soft bristled toothbrush twice a day, both in the morning and at bedtime.
- Clean between the teeth to remove plaques.
- Do not chew tobacco.
- Whenever, first sign of disease occur, consult the doctor.

Joint Problems

Osteoarthritis is common in old age. In a diabetic, this degenerative disorder can be more common and can occur at an earlier age and be more severe. The joints become stiff, painful with restricted mobility. This may result in deformities and the formation of contractures as a result of thickened and contracted tendons and ligaments around the joints. Joints of hands and feet may be affected. However, affliction of the knee joints is common and osteoarthritis of knee joint is by far the most distressing. Surgery involving knee-joint replacement is often contemplated in such cases.

Painkillers are taken frequently to get relief. Those drugs that are toxic to the kidneys should be avoided, such as non-steroidal anti-inflammatory drugs. **Regular** and **proper exercises** designed for each joint is advocated.

Lactic Acidosis

Lactic acidosis is a complication that needs immediate hospitalisation for if left untreated it may prove fatal. One of the most common symptoms is labored breathing. Other symptoms are dizziness, weakness, discomfort, muscle cramps, irregular pulse and feeling cold. Lactic acidosis develops when there is build up of this compound in the blood. Whatever lactic acid is formed in the body it is metabolized in the liver and kidneys. Tendency to develop this complication occurs in patients with compromised liver or kidney functions. Patients with congestive cardiac failure are also at risk.

There are three acute complications of diabetes which may lead to coma, require immediate attention and may require hospitalization.

Hypoglycemia

In hypoglycemia, the blood sugar level falls below 60 mg % or 3.3 mmol per dl or less. The patient feels extreme hunger, anxiety, palpitation, pallor and cold clammy sweating. These symptoms are due to the secretion of **adrenalin**, which comes into action whenever the blood glucose falls. The patient may also feel dizzy, experience loss of concentration, confusion, fatigue and headache. If not corrected it leads to convulsions and coma. This occurs due to inadequate permeation of glucose into the brain cells-neuroglycopenic symptoms. This condition is often precipitated by excessive intake of insulin, oral hypoglycemic drugs as sulphonylureas, inadequate food intake, strenous exercise, alcohol consumption, onset of menses and in the immediate postpartum period. This occurs in a diabetic, who ventures on rigid control of his condition by over exercising and cutting down on his food intake without adequately adjusting the dose of his antidiabetic drugs. Aspirin and other salicylates can also lead to hypoglycemia by potentiating the effect of antidiabetic drugs.

To correct this state, patient must eat candy, or sugar cubes, or drink sugary soft drinks such as orange juice. If patient does not respond to these measures, he should be taken to the hospital. It is advised that all patients of diabetes must carry a candy with them, whenever they go out, to deal with the dangerous situation of hypoglycemia.

Diabetic Ketoacidosis

It is another medical emergency that requires immediate attention. This complication occurs more often in type 1diabetes as compared to type 2, where there is poor control of the disease and inadequate intake of insulin. As a result, there is impaired utilization of glucose, which continues to accumulate in the blood while the tissues are starved. As a corrective reaction, there is increased synthesis of glucose and production of ketone bodies by the liver from fatty acids, which are brought to it from adipose tissue. The ketone bodies accumulate in the blood causing ketosis. The secretion of excess ketones in the urine causes ketonuria. Hyperglycemia results in the loss of sugar in urine, which due to osmosis causes **polyuria** and **dehydration**. Other neurological and gastrointestinal symptoms result from the lack of glucose utilization by brain and gastrointestinal tract.

It is a serious medical emergency and requires immediate hospitalization. However, it is always helpful to understand and know certain aspects of corrective measures. In this condition, it is required to restore the water and electrolyte balance to normal. The potassium and water depletion has to be corrected and insulin has to be given to correct hyperglycemia. As patients vomit, fluids with salts and insulin are given intravenously in the form of a drip, with constant monitoring of blood glucose and electrolyte levels. This is characterized by hyperglycemia, dehydration, ketosis and electrolyte imbalance with potassium deficiency.

Precipitating factors include any other illness, especially an infection, emotional stress and inadequate therapy or new onset of diabetes.

The symptoms of diabetic ketoacidosis include polyuria, polyphagia and polydipsia, headache, malaise, weakness, lethargy, blurred vision, abdominal pain, nausea, vomiting and diarrhoea.

Labored breathing with fruity breath, below normal body temperature and signs of dehydration.

Hyperglycemic, Hyperosmolar, Non Ketotic Syndrome

This complication often occurs in NIDDM elderly patients, taking **oral hypoglycemic drugs**, where the treatment has been inadequate and the disease has not been monitored accurately. The symptoms are same as in the previous condition except for milder gastrointestinal symptoms such as vomiting and diarrhoea and absence of labored breathing. Infections can also precipitate this condition. As in the previous condition, the patient needs to be treated in the hospital and the same corrective measures are to be taken.

Diabetic coma is a medical emergency that requires immediate hospitalization.

---

* Atrophy means destruction or loss of tissue.

PART - III

Prevention, Management & Newer Innovations

Chapter 13

Prevention of Diabetes

"What we think, we become."
Gautam Buddha

In this chapter, an attempt is made to discuss the necessary measures one can possibly take to prevent diabetes. The seeds of diabetes are sown in genes and destiny determines a lot. Yet, certain measures are within our means and we can endeavor to delay or prevent the manifestation of diabetes.

An overview of the Diabetic Prevention Programs initiated and designed by NIH is given in this chapter. Also, a point based system formulated to determine the risk of diabetes and research on Pima Indians and its outcome is mentioned. Drugs and lifestyle changes needed for the prevention of diabetes are discussed.

Disease drains energy. The secret to health lies in prevention of disease. If you are at high risk of developing diabetes, every effort should be made to delay or prevent the onset of the disease. A simple measure is to get your blood sugar tested on regular basis and detect impaired glucose tolerance as early as possible. It is a healthy habit to get yearly check-ups done, especially of blood pressure, blood sugar and serum cholesterol. This is with respect to type 2diabetes, which is much more common than type 1diabetes. Another recommendation is watch your weight.

Onset of Diabetes

One must wake up when the disease is in its dormant phase. One can also call it as a pre-diabetic stage. At this stage, patient may show impaired glucose tolerance (IGT). Otherwise, the disease may spin out of control and precipitate blindness or even amputation of the limbs. This is the time to sit back and ponder on the state of one's physique and take into account one's body weight and lifestyle. This is the time to introspect, think deep and visualize what life will be once the disease strikes. Imagine the restrictions and the complications that might occur, from blindness to amputation. How much one has to pay for the rest of the life in return for a short period of indulgence? It is high time you take control of your life and set your mind to focus on things that are really important and vital to you.

Can we Prevent Diabetes?

Prevention of type 1diabetes is not so easy, as the roots of the malady are ingrained in the person's genetic make up. However, considerable efforts are being made in this direction.

- **Diabetes Prevention Program (DPP),** a body sponsored by NIH (National Institute of Health), has been designed to initiate research and define measures to deal with this major health problems.
- **Two major primary-prevention trials,** in collaboration with NIDDK (National Institute for Diabetes, Digestive and Kidney Diseases) and NIH with the help of private sectors, have been found in late 1990s and the work is in progress. The first trial, the Diabetes Prevention Trial-Type 1(DPT-1) is a national program, designed to study the possibility of preventing or delaying the onset of type 1diabetes. In a number of screening centers relatives of patients, suffering from type 1diabetes, will be investigated for the immunological markers and antibodies involved in the immune destruction of beta cells of the pancreas. If antibodies and beta cell damage is found, the individuals may be put on insulin injections.

Prevention of type 2diabetes is a different situation. If you are overweight and belong to the vulnerable group, then you can do a lot.

The second major prevention trial is the Diabetic Prevention Program. This is also a national study designed to seek individuals at high risk and prevent or delay the development of type 2diabetes by drugs, diet and exercise. Research concerning genetic, metabolic and behavioral risk factors is reviewed and integrated into a comprehensive model of causation and preventive measures are proposed. Their landmark research and findings in a study trial of people with IGT demonstrate that lifestyle intervention and medicine can reduce the risk of developing type 2diabetes. Dr. Sherwin, a professor of medicine at Yale University and former President of the American Diabetes Association states that **"Screening People for IGT does cost money. But, we may able to stave off an epidemic of diabetes which is going to cost us a fortune in a long run, and it may very well be worth the effort".** The results translated to 58% reduction in diabetes risk with lifestyle intervention as compared to 31% with medicine.

Risk factors as overweight and sedentary life style are potentially reversible risk factors. Lifestyle intervention worked across all age, race, and gender groups but was more effective in older people. Potential risk factors as obesity and sedentary life-style are reversible and effective in curbing the incidence of diabetes in high-risk individuals. As reviewed by Anne Maclennan in the New England Journal of Medicine, 7% weight loss and 150 minutes of physical activity per week reduced the incidence by 58% as compared to medicine, where the decrease in incidence was 31%.

Table 13.1 Assessment of Risk for Diabetes and Cardiovascular Disease

S.No.	Risk Factors		Points
1.	Age	35-44 years	8
		45-54 years	18
		55 or older	25
2.	Parent or sibling with heart attack		4
3.	Parent or sibling with diabetes		4
4.	Fasting blood sugar of 110 mg/dl/more		17
5.	Systolic blood pressure of 160mm Hg / more or diastolic blood pressure of 90 mm Hg/ more		10
6.	HDL cholesterol of 35 mg/dl or less		8
7.	Triglycerides of 150 mg/dl		10
8.	Overweight for height (see table 13.2)		10
*	Overweight for height (weight more than the specified range)		21

A point-based system has been formulated for computing an individual's risk of developing diabetes and cardiovascular disease based on data collected at San Antonio Heart Study. **Kenneth L. Williams** presented the model at the annual scientific session of the American Diabetic Association. This model uses eight factors that together can total risk scores that range from 0-100.

Table 13.2 Specified Range of Height and Weight Relationship

S. No.	Height	Overweight
1	5' 0"	128-153 pounds
2	5' 2"	136-164 pounds
3	5' 5"	150-180 pounds
4	5' 8"	164-197 pounds
5	5' 11"	179-215 pounds
6	6' 2"	194-233 pounds

Source: Kenneth L.Williams, San Antonio Heart Study

A person with a score of 20 has about 5% risk of diabetes over the next 8 years. A score of 50 is linked to 40% risk, a score of 65 to 68% risk, a score of 80 to 88% risk and a score of 100 is associated with the maximum risk of 95%.

Obesity: A Prime Cause of Disease

NIDDK has conducted research on Pima Indians for the past 30 years. This research has helped scientists to prove that obesity is a major risk factor in the development of diabetes. About 50% percent of adult Pima Indians are diabetics and 95% of these are overweight. Before gaining weight, these individuals were shown to have lower metabolic rate as compared to non-diabetic adults of similar weight. Slower metabolic rate, high intake of fats combined with the greater tendency to retain fat is responsible for the high incidence of obesity among Pima Indians.

Researchers have used the **"thrifty gene"** theory proposed in 1962 by geneticist James Neel, to explain the overweight epidemic seen in Pima Indians. The Neel's theory is based on the population studies of those communities, who relied on farming, hunting and fishing for their daily food needs, for thousands of years. These people faced alternating periods of feast and famine. Neel said that to adapt to these extreme changes in calorie needs, these people developed a thrifty gene, which allowed them to store food in times of plenty so that they would not starve in time of need. But once these people shifted and adopted the Western lifestyle, with less physical activity, excess intake of fatty food and access to constant supply of calories, the gene worked against them, and these people continued to store excess fat. Dr Ravussin says that the only way to correct obesity is to eat less fat and exercise regularly.

Greater Risk Category

Anyone can develop diabetes but certain individuals are more at risk than others. Persons at greater risk have following characteristics:

- With positive family history of diabetes.
- Who are 40 years of age or older.
- Who are overweight, especially with localization of excess fat in the upper part of abdomen, chest, neck and face. The waist to hip ratio is more than 0.9 in men and 0.8 in women.
- Women who had diabetes during pregnancy or delivered a baby nine pounds or more in weight.
- People with high blood pressure or high blood lipid level.
- Children born to diabetic mothers are at greater risk in becoming obese and developing diabetes.
- Persons belonging to the high risk ethnic group as African American, Hispanic, Native American, and Asian.
- Impaired glucose tolerance on any previous testing.

Such persons can prevent or at least delay the onset of diabetes by weight reduction, regulating their diet, drastically reducing consumption of alcoholic drinks, and doing regular exercise. *If the person is just overweight then the risk factor is 10. However, if the overweight is more than the specified range then the risk factor becomes 21. They must also get their blood sugar, blood lipid and blood pressure checked regularly.

Precautions for Risk Category

It is now believed that every individual who is thirty years of age or over must get his blood sugar and lipid profile done regularly. This is to detect diabetes in its insipient or pre-diabetic stage. This is more so for individuals at greater risk. As the incidence of diabetes is on the rise, these measures will diminish the morbidity.

Pregnant women with average risk of diabetes should be screened between 24 and 28 weeks of gestation. Those women who are 25 years or older and with high risk factors should undergo glucose testing as early as possible and then between 24 and 28 weeks of gestation.

Some research investigations and preliminary data suggest that higher intake of omega-3 fatty acids, present in fish, might protect people from developing type 2 DM.

Drugs that lower blood lipids, as cholesterol, triglycerides and LDL also help in decreasing the mortality and morbidity in persons with impaired glucose tolerance and those with type 2diabetes.

Chapter 14

LET NOT OUR CHILDREN HAVE DIABETES

Are the children at greater risk of developing diabetes? Are the alarm bells ringing? These questions should haunt the minds of parents, teachers and administrators alike.

Type 1diabetes in Children

Children generally suffer from type 1diabetes. Every year about 13000 new cases of type 1diabetes are diagnosed. Researchers have made some progress in depicting who is at risk for developing this variant of diabetes. However, scientists have not been able to unravel what triggers the onset of the disease. It is believed that it is the combination of genetic and environmental factors. Efforts are directed towards identifying the external agent that precipitates the disease. Perhaps a viral infection is responsible for the initiation of lethal attack on insulin producing cells of pancreas. Research is directed to identify the external source that initiates the autoimmune attack on beta cells of pancreas, resulting in almost complete loss of synthesis of insulin.

Type 2diabetes in Children

However, at present the incidence of type 2diabetes in children is gradually creeping up and gaining momentum. Type 2diabetes is linked to obesity and insulin resistance. Type 2diabetes affects children, teens and adults. Detecting type 2diabetes in children can be difficult as children may have no or mild symptoms and unless blood tests are carried out, diagnosis cannot be established. According to Disease Control and Prevention's statistics, the incidence of type 2diabetes in children and adolescents in North America is generally in the age group 16 and 19 years of age. All ethnic groups suffer but American Indian youth have the highest prevalence.

Obesity and Diabetes

These children are obese, insulin resistant and have strong family history of diabetes. Those children, who lost 5% of their body weight, reduced the risk of disease by 61% (New England Journal of Medicine. 344, 1343-1349, 2001).

The rate of obesity among children has increased dramatically over the past two decades, and along with it health problems as high blood pressure, high blood cholesterol and diabetes.

According to the recent survey by CDC, nearly 14% of students are overweight in the state of Arkansas, (Washington Post, August 20, 2003). About 15% of US children are overweight, according to the Centers for Disease Control and Prevention in Atlanta. **"Overweight children developing chronic diseases, that will plague them for life**, including **Type 2diabetes**, is a growing problem among children that is triggered by excessive weight and inactivity," as per Washington Post.

Table 14.1 Percentage of overweight students.

State	Overweight %
Texas	14.2%
Mississippi	14%
North Carolina	12.9%
Missouri	12.8%

Source: Youth Risk Behavior Survey; 2001,CDC

Responsibility of Parents

The morning starts with cola and the day ends with cola, while it should start with a glass of clean, clear water and end with water. Then drive down to fast food shop, sitting in the car with mom and pop, buy a big hamburger, come home, eat sitting in front of the TV. This is the worst you can do to your kid.

Children are innocent and they do not know what is right for them. It is the responsibility of parents to inculcate **healthy eating habits** in their kids. It is sad and unfortunate that the very hands that nurture and protect them, groom and breed them are responsible for leading them on a path of indulgence and malady.

Precautions During Childhood

Children present unique opportunity in the field of preventive maneuvers. Avoiding initial excess weight gain can prevent obesity and secondary prevention by stopping further gain while the child grows and the weight gets adjusted naturally. Understanding the origin of obesity is important as it helps to formulate correct strategies. It has been found that children predisposed to type 2diabetes have generally low birth weight and are thin in infancy. They tend to gain weight rapidly in early childhood and become obese in adolescence.

It has been reported that even a mild increase in BMI in childhood increases the risk of diabetes manifold. "The association of adult obesity and its complications with birth weight, rebound of the BMI and overweight during adolescence, suggests that these periods may prove critical for the prevention of early overweight and its effect on adult disease" Dr William H Dietz-from Center for Disease Control and Prevention in Atlanta.

If a whole generation of diabetic children is allowed to grow, the cost in terms of health care and lost hours of manpower will run into billions of dollars.

Today's concerns about childhood obesity have created the need for better understanding about the eating habits of children. Research has shed light on the eating habits of children. An 8-year study from the University of Tennessee has shown that the babies' food habits developed in the first two years of life influence its habits later on in life. Hence, the first two years are critical in initiating healthy food choices, adequate nutritional intake and exposure to right amount of calorie intake.

Some Considerable Facts

- Colas are rich in non-nutritive calories and put extra calorie load on the body.
- Develop the habit of giving children three major healthy nutritive meals and only healthy snacks in between such as peanuts or almonds. Do not force the child to eat unless hungry. When body needs food the hunger bells ring and the body gives signals such as emptiness in the pit of stomach.
- Avoid excess candy and desserts. Further, as children spend lot of time in schools, policies adopted in schools should promote physical activities.
- Expose toddlers and children to healthy food choices. It has been reported that developing the habit of eating generous amounts of fruits and vegetables in early life enhances the chances of taking more fruits and vegetables later in life.

"The number of older infants and toddlers who are not consuming vegetables is striking. Among 9-11 month olds, 27% consumed no separate serving of vegetable in a day, and among toddlers older than 12 months, between 18-23% did not consume vegetables.

A study published in "Journal of the American Dietetic Association, 104 (1) 2004" states that Nutrition experts have shown that eating different colored fruits and vegetables provide different phytonutrients, which have various health benefits.

Chapter 15

Management of Diabetes

This chapter is divided into three sections and many aspects about care of feet, exercise and food are discussed.

1st section deals with the care of feet and general hygiene.

2nd section about various types of exercises-yogic, aerobic and anaerobic. Stress is laid on the benefit and need for the exercise. The amount of exercise and calories burnt thereby is tabulated.

3rd part deals about ideal body weight, need to lose weight where required, calorie intake, foods with their nutrient value, type of food to be eaten and balanced sensible food plan.

A great scientist announced that gene proposes and environment disposes. In other words, environment exposes what we inherit. How much of the environment can be handled depends, to quite an extent, on our own activities. At this point. I am reminded of a narration from the epic of Mahabharta.

"This is your *karm bhoomi*".

The ancient Indian epic, the Mahabharata epitomizes and immortalizes it through an engrossing narration of events- clash of ambitions, spiraling greed, a chain of deceptions, gambles, and finally this culminates in a bloody battle on the fields of *Kurukshetra*. But not before the Lord's incarnation Krishna, unveils the essence of man's existence, his spiritual nature, the ethos of religious philosophy and the laws of karma to his wavering warrior-disciple *Arjun*.

As the story unfolds, the ruling monarch and uncle of *Pandavs*, split the kingdom of *Hastinapur*, which rightly belonged to the *Pandavs*. While the flourishing, bountiful chunk was gifted to the monarch's eldest son, a small piece of barren land was given to the *Pandavs*.

When the despairing *Pandavs* turned to Lord Krishna, they were told – "This is your *Karam bhoomi*" meaning from this land you carve out your destiny by your deeds *Karma* means deed/action and *Bhoomi* means land."

Diabetes is Mainly a Self-managed Condition

Management and treatment of type 1diabetes is different from type 2. Although, the principal goal is to achieve blood glucose levels within normal limits, in all types of diabetes, yet other factors greatly modify the treatment. Age, sex, working circumstances, overall health status and life style influence the management objectives. Requirements in young growing children differ from those in elderly adults. Similarly, the demands in middle-aged working women are different. Pregnancy and menstrual cycle pose their own challenges. "When to eat, how much to eat, type of food, dose of medicine, amount and type of exercise vary from person to person."

Treatment goals have to be tailored according to individual demands.

Regime and Treatment of Individual Demands

The treatment of diabetes requires management of multiple aspects of this disease. It is not just the education of the patient, but also of his relatives so that diabetes management becomes a team effort, who take part in a multi-disciplinary approach in care of the patient. Acute and chronic hazards of the disease should be recognized early and treated as soon as possible to prevent irreversible damage. An overenthusiastic approach in the treatment regime and attempt to achieve normal blood glucose level, may cause **hypoglycemia** that is low blood glucose levels especially when the patient is taking insulin. Such episodes occur more often in type 1diabetes, as the patient is totally dependent on insulin for the management of his disease.

Hypoglycemia

It is a life threatening condition and the patient must be fully aware of the symptoms. The symptoms may be due to impaired functions of the brain such as dizziness, mental confusion, bizarre behavior, or fainting leading to **coma**. Hypoglycemia causes reactionary secretion of hormones such as adrenalin (secreted by the adrenal gland, which is situated above the kidney) to raise glucose levels in the body. Symptoms due to the action of adrenalin may dominate the picture. These are palpitation, (awareness of heartbeat), sweating, tachycardia, which means increased heart rate, and tremors. Patient may experience extreme hunger and are advised to carry with them some candy or sugar tablet or drink orange juice if it is available. Elderly diabetics should not try to attempt very tight control of their disease. Such episodes of hypoglycemia may precipitate a **heart attack**.

Care of Feet

Care of the feet is essential and cannot be overemphasized as neglect of feet can cause morbidity and even mortality. Feet should be washed daily with soap and water. These should be dried, especially between the toes and not rubbed too vigorously, to avoid cracks in the delicate skin. After drying, rub vegetable oil or moisturizer into the feet to keep them soft and prevent cracks and dryness. Do not walk barefoot. Moreover, the shoes should never be tight. These should be wide, have low heels, must be well fitting, comfortable, and preferably leather made. Feet should be inspected daily for any cuts or abrasions and if there are any, should be treated immediately. Any red or blue patch on the feet should be given immediate attention. Do not cut corns on the feet. Cut the toe nails straight and avoid cutting the corners of the toe nails. If the feet tend to remain moist and there are chances of developing fungal infections, then it is advisable to use dusting powder.

Many diabetic patients have cold feet due to vascular and circulatory disturbances. In such situations, patient could take certain precautions. Wear warm stockings, as cold constricts the blood vessels further and avoid circular garters. These compress the vessels and further impair the circulation.

Completely avoid **tobacco** in any form, as tobacco contract the blood vessels and decrease circulation. Hot water pads and heat should be avoided, as this tends to burn the delicate skin. If ulcer develops, it should be treated under medical supervision. Ulcer, if neglected can get infected leading to a non-healing wound, which may subsequently result in amputation. The ulcer area should be kept relaxed, elevated and free of pressure, as these measures help in the healing process. A number of ointments that promote healing are available in the market. These should be used after medical considerations.

Always Rembember

- Stop smoking.
- Do not walk barefooted even at home.
- Inspect the feet daily for any cuts or abrasions.
- Shake out the shoes before wearing them.
- Wear porous, clean, cotton or woolen socks.
- Do feet and leg exercises daily.
- Keep feet clean, dry with the application of moisturizer in between toes.
- In the event of an ulcer or non-healing wound, consult the doctor.
- Feet should be the cleanest part of the body.

Precautionary Measures

A diabetic should strictly follow certain precautionary measures. Some of them are discussed here in this section.

Diet Management

"While we need so little to survive, we need so much to appease our appetites." No doubt there were those who thought Hippocrates was behind the times in 400 B.C, when the father of modern medicine said:

"Let food be your medicine and medicine be your food". But he was a visionary who thought ahead of his times, as diet management is the key to diabetes control. **Thomas Edison**, the inventing visionary, claimed that the doctor of the future will not give medicine but will interest his patient in the care of human frame in diet and in the care of disease.

Meal planning and diet regulation is crucial in controlling diabetes. Various aspects of diet need to be managed. **A well-balanced, nutritious diet is required in all types of diabetes**. However, the stress is laid on different aspects in different situations. Diet has to be tailored on individual basis depending on metabolic rate and life style requirements. In obese, type 2diabetes stress is focused on weight reduction. In such patients, intake of carbohydrates and fats has to be reduced. Also, portion of carbohydrates are to be substituted by monounsaturated non-cholesterologenic fats such as olive oil and rapeseed oil (canola). This also applies to patient in whom it is difficult to get good glycemic control, especially type 1diabetes, who are on insulin therapy.

It is recommended that in all types of diabetes, the total cholesterol content should not exceed 300 mg per day. The total protein content should constitute 10-20% of daily calorie intake, the monounsaturated fats should form about 10 % and polyunsaturated form another 10% of daily calorie intake. The saturated fats are to be discouraged in all individuals. Part of treatment of type 2diabetes is weight reduction. Losing weight means eating less and eating less means fewer intake of calories. Fats are the most concentrated form of calories. So best way to accomplish weight loss is to cut down on fats especially saturated fats.

Body Weight

An ideal body weight is the first pre-requisite for good health but for a diabetic it is absolutely essential. If type 2diabetes is associated with obesity, the first line of management is weight reduction. The weight reduction and diet control may be sufficient to manage type 2diabetes.

It is beneficial to shed extra pounds for good body weight control. It helps to prevent the progression of impaired glucose tolerance to type 2diabetes. It also helps to reverse the failure to respond to drugs. It reduces blood pressure, improves lipid profile and reduces the risk of death from the complications of diabetes. In determining the calorie needs of the body, it is necessary to know the ideal body weight. The weight-height tables for men and women for three body frame sizes are given below.

Table 15.1 Height-Weight relation in men between 25-59 years of age.

Height	Weight in pounds		
	Small Frame	Medium Frame	Large Frame
5'2"	128-134	131-141	138-150
5'3"	130-136	133-143	140-153
5'4"	132-138	135-145	142-156
5'5"	134-140	137-148	144-160
5'6"	136-142	139-151	146-164
5'7"	138-145	142-154	152-172
5'8"	140-148	145-157	152-176
5'9"	142-151	148-160	158-180
5'10'	144-154	151-163	158-180
5'11"	146-157	154-166	161-184
6'0"	149-160	157-170	164-188
6'1"	152-164	160-174	168-192
6'2"	155-164	164-178	172-197
6'3"	158-172	167-182	176-202
6'4"	162-176	171-187	181-207

Table 15.2 Height-Weight relation in women between 25-50 years of age.

Height	Weight in pounds		
	Small Frame	Medium Frame	Large Frame
4'10"	102-111	109-121	118-131
4'11"	103-113	111-123	120-134
5'0"	104-115	113-126	122-137
5'1"	106-118	115-129	125-140
5'2"	108-121	118-132	128-143
5'3"	111-124	121-135	131-147
5'4"	114-127	124-138	134-151
5'5"	117-130	127-147	137-155
5'6"	120-133	130-144	140-159
5'76"	123-136	133-147	143-163

5'8"	126-139	136-150	146-167
5'9"	129-142	139-153	149-170
5'10"	132-145	142-156	152-173
5'11"	135-148	145-159	155-176
6'0"	138-151	148-162	158-179

Source: The Metropolitan Life Insurance Company (1983).

A simple formula to calculate ideal body weight is:

Man – 50 kg for first 5' + 2.3 kg for each 1" over 5'

Woman – 45.5 kg for first 5' + 2.3 kg for each 1" over 5'

An obese person is one who weighs 20% more than the ideal body weight.

Calorie Requirement

Total calorie content taken daily varies from person to person depending on age, sex, height, metabolic rate and life style requirement. Minimum daily requirement is 10 calories per pound of **ideal body weight**. This means that if the person's ideal weight is 150 pounds then his basic requirement is 1500 calories per day. To this basic need, additional calories are added depending on the degree of activity. For a person, leading sedentary life an additional 10% of basal calorie requirement, for a person with moderate activity, an additional 20% and for active life, 40% or more is needed. For example, a person with ideal body weight of 150 pounds and leading a moderately active life needs 1500 calories plus 20% of 1500, which is 300 calories totaling to 1800 calories. Thus, a person about 50 years of age, doing light to moderate activity requires an additional 300 calories per day. A young person engaged in vigorous daily routine needs about 1000 or more calories in addition to the basic recommended intake, i.e. 2500-3000 calories per day. A diabetic woman who is pregnant or lactating, likewise needs additional about 1000 or more calories. In case of attempts at trying to lose weight, the number of calories consumed must correspondingly decrease. For no matter what is said, the body weight is determined by the number of calories eaten minus the number of calories burned by the activity.

One gram of protein and one gram of carbohydrate yield 4 calories, whereas one gram of alcohol gives 7 calories and one gram of fat burns to give 9 calories. After determining the calorie requirement, the meals of the day can be planned.

Dietary Fiber

Dietary fibers should constitute an important portion of the daily food intake. There are two types of fibers, soluble and insoluble found in foods. The insoluble fibers are **cellulose** and **hemicellulose**. These are found in bran and green leafy vegetables as spinach, mustard leaves, cabbage and lettuce. As these are not absorbed from the intestinal tract they help to form bulk of the waste that collects in the large intestine, which is necessary for the optimal intestinal motility. Optimal intestinal motility is required for the healthy colonic functions and prevents stagnation of food residues in the gut. This minimizes contact of harmful ingredients such as carcinogens with the wall of colon and reduces absorption of food articles in the diet such as cholesterol.

The soluble fibers, which include gums and pectin's, are found in oatmeal, apple, and beans. These retard the rate of absorption of nutrients, thereby diminishing the incidence of rapid rise of blood sugar level at meals. These also lower LDL cholesterol in blood and increase HDL cholesterol. As the saying goes, **"an apple a day keeps the doctor away."** Vegetarian diet is better than non-vegetarian diet for more than one reason.

Vegetarian diet is obtained from plants, which include cereals, lentils, beans, fruits and vegetables. It is rich in fiber content. These foods contain complex carbohydrates and they have polyunsaturated and monounsaturated fats. The non-vegetarian diet, obtained from animals, includes red meat, poultry, milk and milk products and contains very high content of saturated fats, no fiber, and simple sugars that are rapidly absorbed and raise blood glucose level. Hence, a vegetarian diet is highly recommended in diabetic patient. Diet should have 30-40 grams of fibers per day.

Water

A lot is written about the food we eat. Much is discussed about the different types of food. No doubt food is important, but no less important is the water we drink. Adequate water must be consumed each day. This is important for optimal kidney and bowel functions. It is also required for fully hydrated healthy skin, which excretes sweat along with some body waste and helps to maintain the body temperature. Water and air are vital to life. The air we breathe and the water we drink are the two most important elements required for all living beings. Pure and clean water is essential for healthy living. Drinking bottled water is a possible alternative, but one has to be sure of the source. Many a time, the bottled water is simply repackaged pipeline supply. Drinking filtered water is another possible option, especially in the third world countries where drinking water supplied in the pipeline is of questionable purity and therefore, filtered water is a more reliable one. There are many types of water filters installed in homes for domestic uses. Most of these filters, if obtained from the standard manufacturers and if regularly serviced, are good enough. Most of these filters use **carbon block** filtration that remove organic chemicals, and **reverse osmosis**, which is effective against inorganic pollutants like lead and nitrates; deionization resins achieve the same objective.

Microwater

A new water filtration method, originally developed in Japan, is a system to form **microwater**. This is a technology where water is filtered and the size of the water molecules is made smaller. A small electrical charge is ejected through the water and this separates water into two types, acidic water and alkaline water. **Acidic water** is used for external and topical purposes and alkaline water for drinking purposes. According to recent research, the acidic water is a super-oxidant and can disinfect and sterilize surfaces. Besides bathing, washing fruits and vegetables, cleaning dishes, it has been used to clean wounds and even disinfect surgical instruments. Acidic water can kill bacteria and viruses.

According to Dr. Hayashi, M.D., one of the Japans foremost Microwater researchers, the alkaline water is a powerful antioxidant similar to vitamins A, C and E. Like other antioxidants, this water destroys all harmful free radicals liberated in the body during metabolism. As the size of a water molecule is smaller, it can penetrate the cells and tissues more effectively, deliver the nutrients to the cells and remove the waste better. According to Dr. Hayashi, those who have been **drinking microwater** every day for several months have shown improvement in their status of diabetes, blood pressure, allergies, obesity, osteoporosis, and some other irregularities. Some firms in California are producing such microwater units that can be easily installed in homes. This alkaline water tastes like mountain spring water. For more details on the subject of microwater, refer to- Definitive Guide to Cancer by: W. John Diamond, M.D., W. Lee Cowden, M.D., with, Burton Goldberg, Future Medicine Publishing, Inc., Tiburon, California.

Proteins

Proteins in our diet constitute an important and essential ingredient. On an average, a man requires a minimum of 50 grams and a woman a minimum of 40 grams of protein per day. Growing children, pregnant and lactating mothers require an extra 15-20 grams of protein per day, not exceeding 15% of total calorie intake.

Persons engaged in active physical labor, do not need extra intake of proteins if calorie intake in the form of carbohydrates and fats is adequate. Proteins are essential for the growth and maintenance of tissues because they constitute an integral part of the tissues, especially muscles. Also, proteins are required for the synthesis of hormones and enzymes. Amino acids are the building blocks of proteins and most of these can be synthesized in the body when required. There are about nine essential amino acids, which cannot be manufactured by the body and need to be consumed in our food. Proteins obtained from animal source such as poultry, fish and dairy products are rich in essential amino acids, whereas proteins obtained from plant source lack one or more of the essential amino acids.

It is recommended that at least 50% of protein intake should be from animal source to ensure adequate supply of essential amino acids in diet. With wear and tear of the tissues, amino acids are lost from the body and therefore these amino acids, present in proteins, need to be replenished in the diet. Among the amino acids, proline and lysine are important building blocks of collagen fiber, which are required to preserve the stability of the blood vessel wall.

Plant Proteins

The **plant proteins** present in cereals, beans and lentils are considered a good source of amino acids. The proteins found in soybeans are highly concentrated. Soybeans also contain phytoestrogen and isoflavones, which are said to decrease the incidence of cancer of the prostate gland in men and cancer of the breast in women. Other beans also contain phytoestrogen and also help in reducing menopausal symptoms.

Animal Proteins

An egg has more than 200 mgs of cholesterol in egg yolk and is considered unhealthy. Fish food is regarded among the best form of proteins from the animal source as besides proteins, it also contains oil rich in vitamins and omega 3-fatty acids, which is good for the heart. Omega 3-fatty acids are long chain polyunsaturated fatty acids that help to increase the HDL cholesterol level in blood, which is protective in nature. The Eskimos consume lot of fat in the form of fish oils but remain at lower risk for cancer and heart disease. Among the fish mackerel, sardines and herring are considered better sources of omega 3-fatty acids, which have three double bonds. Too much of protein however, is bad for health. The excess proteins are lost in urine thereby overloading the kidneys. Also, the amino acids remove calcium from the bones while these are excreted. This leads to osteoporosis.

Carbohydrate Intake and Vigil

Carbohydrates are required to provide energy in the body. About 55-65 % of calorie intake should be in the form of carbohydrates. Carbohydrates are classified into, simple as sugars and complex as starch. A diabetic patient should always avoid intake of sugars. Not only do they constitute a concentrated form of calories, but they also lack in nutrients and their consumption rapidly raises blood glucose levels. They also cause tooth decay. Complex carbohydrates found in cereals, lentils, legumes and beans are highly recommended, as they are rich in fibers and other nutrients. The cereals include wheat, oat, barley, and rice and need to be taken as whole and not in the refined form, otherwise the fiber content is lost. Oats are beneficial as they lower LDL cholesterol and raise HDL cholesterol. **Barley i**s considered even better in this respect.

Artificial Sweeteners

The role of sweeteners in a diabetic needs to be reviewed. There are natural sugars as sucrose or cane sugar and artificial sweeteners.

Sugars have no nutritive value, they only add to calories. The continuous use of these substances continues to increase the desire for sweets. Foods with high content of sugars impair glucose control and should be eaten sparingly. The desire for sweets should be mitigated at all costs in a diabetic.

Artificial sweeteners as **saccharin** and **aspartames** have no calorie value. Some of these compounds were considered carcinogenic, but now it is agreed that these compounds were found to be carcinogenic in animal experiments only. "But if you need to control your sugar and calorie intake, artificial sweeteners are safe, and effective way to do so," said Ruth Kava, Director of nutrition for the American Council on Science and Health.

FDA has given its approval for the following five artificial sweeteners now available in the market.

1. Aspartame (Nutra sweet or Equal)
2. Acesulfame potassium (Sunett)
3. D-Tagatose (Sugaree)
4. Sucralose (Splenda)
5. Saccharin (Sweet N low). This compound was introduced in 1879 and it is 300 times sweeter than sugar.

The herbal sweetener called **Stevia** has been in use by South American natives for many centuries and in Japan since mid 1970s.

Natural Sweeteners

Natural sweeteners such as **sorbitol** and **fructose** have become popular as effective sweetening agents. These may cause diarrhea as a side effect. Taken in high doses these tend to raise LDL cholesterol. However, taken in fruits and taken in small amounts, these are not harmful. But, a diabetic should always exercise restraint and eat in moderation.

The US Food and Drug Administration, has most recently given approval to a new nonnutritive sweetener, **sucralose**, derived from table sugar, for use in food products. It is believed to be 600 times as sweet as sugar.

Fatty Alarm

Fats are the richest and the most concentrated source of energy in food. Besides, fats are tasty and give a sense of satiety; hence people tend to consume an increased quantity of fat in their diet. In the body, fats are required to produce energy.

Fats eaten in excess are stored in fat depots and cause obesity with all the harmful consequences. Extra calories taken that are not burned down also get stored in the form of fat. Nature created fat as food reserve in the body but if the boundary is crossed the result is dangerous. Not more than 35 grams of fat is to be consumed per day and the total calorie intake in the form of fats should not exceed 20%. If, however, the calorie requirement is high, the amount of fat intake may be increased to 45 grams.

Fats taken in meals fall into two categories, **cholesterol** and **fatty acids** with their derivative, the **triglycerides**. Cholesterol is present as a structural component of the cell membrane. The body can easily synthesize it. We do not require any cholesterol from an external source. If we consume cholesterol in our diet, we only raise the cholesterol levels in blood, which is not good for the heart. Fatty acids are either **saturated**, or **unsaturated**.

Saturated Fatty Acids

Saturated fatty acids are said to be associated with increased incidence of heart attack and it is strongly recommended that diets should exclude these types of fatty acids. Foods from animal source such as beef, meat, pork, eggs and chicken are very rich in saturated fatty acids. Fats present in dairy products are also of the same type. Saturated fats are solid at room temperature.

Unsaturated Fatty Acids

The unsaturated fatty acids may be monounsaturated or **polyunsaturated**. It is now recommended that diet should include unsaturated fatty acids, preferably monounsaturated fatty acids, found in olive oil, canola oil, avocados, and complex carbohydrates. Monounsaturated fatty acids are also found in peanuts, pistachio and cashew nuts.

A polyunsaturated fatty acid called **linoleic acid** (found in corn, peanut, walnut, cottonseed oil, soybean and many plant oils) is an essential nutrient and should be present in our meal, as the body cannot synthesize it. Its deficiency causes loss of hair, dermatitis and impaired wound healing. Other essential fatty acids include linolenic acid (found in linseed oil) and arachidonic acid. These are found along with the linoleic acid. These compounds constitute the structural integrity of the cells and occur in high concentration in the reproductive organs. The deficiency of these essential fatty acids in experimental rats, have been shown to cause skin disorders and reproductive deficiency. Unsaturated fats are fluid at room temperature.

Vitamins

Vitamins, minerals and trace metals constitute important ingredients required by the cells. These are needed by the cells to perform their metabolic functions to generate **bioenergy**. Each cell in the body needs energy for its optimum functions. Vitamins are a group of organic compounds that constitute an essential portion of our dietary requirements, as our body cannot synthesize these molecules. They are divided into **water soluble** and **fat-soluble compounds**.

- Water-soluble vitamins include C and B.
- Fat-soluble are A, D, E and K. Vitamins and minerals or the foods containing these nutrients, have been used as therapy for thousands of years.

Scientific research has revealed the significance of vitamins, beta-carotene, lysine, proline, bioflavonoids, carnitine, and coenzyme Q-10 in the prevention of diabetes, hypertension and atherosclerosis.

Need for Vitamins

Dr. Linus Pauling, a two time Nobel laureate, did extensive work in nutritional research and cellular medicine. He advocated that health and disease are determined at cellular levels. The cells require vitamins and other essential nutrients to perform millions of chemical reactions, and deficiency of these ingredients will eventually lead to the malfunctioning of the cells and cause disease. Those organs and systems that work the hardest undergo wear and tear the most and bear a greater brunt of deficiency.

Ancient Egyptians ate the liver of roosters to cure night blindness as these were rich in vitamin A and ate sea sponge, a natural source of iodine to treat goiter. Excess of anything is bad and therefore excess of vitamins and minerals taken in the form of supplements should be discouraged unless prescribed by the doctor. Fat-soluble vitamins, when taken in excess are stored in fat depots in the body while excess of water-soluble vitamins are lost in urine. Vitamins and minerals are crucial to health. They do not release energy but some of them form part of enzymes that help to release energy from fats and carbohydrates. Every cell in the body requires minerals and vitamins in different proportions and for different purposes, e.g. bones and teeth need calcium the most. Some of the important vitamins and their functions are discussed below.

Vitamin A

It is required for the healthy maintenance of skin, lining of body cavities such as oral cavity, stomach, intestine, food pipe and others. It also helps in the growth of bone and teeth. Deficiency of this vitamin can produce **blindness in children**. Vitamin A is thus needed for healthy skin, strong bones, teeth and eyes. It is found in carrots, green leafy vegetables as spinach, broccoli, mangoes, apricots, water melon, cantaloupe, sweet potato and tuna fish. 5000 IU of vitamin A is needed per day.

Vitamin B

Among this group of vitamins, Folic acid, Vitamin B-6 and B-12 are three important nutrients required for the synthesis of red blood cells, which are the carriers of oxygen in the blood. Needless to mention, as life is not possible without oxygen, it is imperative to take adequate amount of these vitamins for the viability of the tissues. It includes the following compounds:

1. **Vitamin B-1** also called **Thiamine**. It is essential for healthy nervous system and carbohydrate metabolism. It functions as a cofactor for pyrophosphate, which acts as a catalyst in carbohydrate metabolism to produce energy bonds required by every cell of the body to perform its functions. Wheat, rice bran, peanuts, legumes, oatmeal, oranges, watermelon and eggs contain it. Daily requirement is 1.5 mg.

2. **Vitamin B-2** also known as **Riboflavin**. It helps in fat, protein and carbohydrate metabolism. It functions as a cofactor for adenine-dinucleotide, which is one of the most important carrier molecules of high-energy bonds in the cells. It is available in dairy products, fish, cereals, mushrooms, turnip, broccoli and turkey. Daily need is 1.7 mg per day.
3. **Vitamin B-3** also called **Niacin**. It is needed in the metabolism of fat, protein and carbohydrates, optimal utilization of oxygen by cells and functional physiology of the nervous system. It is an essential component of nicotinamide-adenine-dinucleotide (NAD), an important carrier of high-energy bonds in the cells power plants. It is found in nature in peanut butter, legumes, soybeans, whole grain cereals, broccoli, meat, poultry and fish. Daily requirement is 20 mg.
4. **Vitamin B-6** also known as **Pyridoxine**. It is required for protein metabolism for normal growth and is essential for strong immunity. It is also needed for the production of red blood cells. The red blood cells transport oxygen in the circulation. It is present in fish, soybean, banana, cauliflower, potato, green pepper, spinach, raisins and chicken. The daily requirement is 2 mg.
5. **Folic acid** is used in the formation of red blood cells, tissue growth and repair. It is found in tuna fish, poultry, wheat, mushroom, banana, strawberry, cantaloupe and oranges. Daily need is 0.4 mg.
6. **Vitamin B-12** is required for the red blood cell formation, optimal function of nervous system and new tissue growth. It is found in salmon, eggs, cheese, tuna, crab, oyster, swordfish and mussel. Daily need is 6 mcg.
7. **Biotin** helps in fat, protein and carbohydrate metabolism. Natural sources of this vitamin are egg, nuts especially peanut, oatmeal, wheat germ, legumes, and cauliflower. The daily requirement is 0.3 mg; higher doses may be given in diabetes.
8. **Vitamin B-5** also called **Pantothenic acid** is used in fat, protein and carbohydrate metabolism. It is a cofactor in acetyl coenzyme A, a key molecule in the production of high-energy bonds. It is

found in fish, whole grain cereals, avocados, peanut, cashew, lentils, soybeans and eggs. Daily need is 10 mg.

9. **Vitamin C** is required in the growth and maintenance of ground substance of the tissues of the body. It is required for the production of collagen fibers, elastic fibers and connective tissue molecules that form the cement to bind tissues and cells together. Just as a building can collapse without cement, same also the cells of the body lose their format without collagen, as in scurvy.

   Thus, this vitamin is needed in the continuous process of repair and regeneration of tissues, which are lost in the wear and tear of the body cells. The abrasions in the vessel wall hold special significance as these predispose to atherosclerosis. It is a strong antioxidant. The rich sources are citrus fruits such as oranges, grapes and vegetables such as cabbage, broccoli, tomatoes, and other fruits as raspberry and strawberry. Daily requirement is 60 mg but 500 -1000 mg is recommended for healing conditions. In diabetics, up to 2000 mg is recommended by some authorities.

   We recommend one should take, if possible 10 to 12 glasses of water with fresh lemon juice, with or without little honey added to it and also offer to guests in every home and office instead of coke, diet or otherwise.

10. **Vitamin D** is needed for the metabolism of calcium and growth and maintenance of bones and teeth. Its rich source is milk and milk products, tuna, salmon, cereals and eggs. Without adequate amount of this vitamin, the growth is retarded and the bones become weak and malformed. Daily requirement is 400 I.U.

11. **Vitamin E** is an **anti-aging vitamin**. It is a strong antioxidant and protects cells from damage. It is also believed to keep the blood thin and less sticky. It is found in nuts as peanuts, wheat germ, mangoes, blackberry, broccoli, spinach and apples. Daily need is 30 I.U. However, in healing conditions up to 400-600 units can be taken.

12. **Vitamin K** is required for the process of blood clotting in the body. It is present in spinach, broccoli, sprouts, cabbage, parsley, carrots, tomatoes and dairy products. Daily requirement is 6 mcg.

Anti Oxidants : The Protective Shield

Antioxidants are substances that neutralize the effects of **free oxygen radicals** and super-oxides or pro-oxidants liberated in the body during metabolic activity and more so during infection and inflammation occurring in any disease process. Free radicals are also increased by the consumption of alcohol and cured meat. Intake of herbicides, asbestos and chemotherapeutic drugs and exposure to ultraviolet rays, X-rays and car exhaust also induce the production of these radicals. Food preservatives, coloring, frying and barbecuing of foods have similar effect. These harmful radicals damage the cells. They induce degeneration in the tissues and enhance the **aging process**. They also act on chromosomal matter of cells and induce carcinogenesis. A pre-requisite for the deposition of LDL cholesterol in the wall of blood vessels is the oxidation of LDL by these radicals, which subsequently leads to **atherosclerosis**. These free radicals can damage the pancreas producing diabetes, and act on lens of the eye, causing cataract. These pro-oxidants also compromise the immune system of the body. The levels of these chemicals are higher in diabetics making them vulnerable to oxidative damage.

Some Antioxidants

Today, the frontline in the treatment of diabetes and other diseases of old age such as cancer and heart disease is the intake of **high doses** of **antioxidants**. Vitamin A, E and C are very good antioxidants. Phytochemicals are powerful and rich sources of antioxidants present in fruits and vegetables such as green leafy vegetables as cabbage, broccoli, carrots, tomatoes, citrus fruits, ginger and garlic. Soy and cereals also have antioxidants. Beverages as tea and coffee, nuts as peanuts, fish and curd containing acidophilus also contain antioxidants. Phytochemicals have strong anticancer activity, retard tumor growth and are powerful inhibitors of breast, colon and prostate cancer. They block the absorption of cholesterol from gut; lower the level of cholesterol in blood, prevent clogging of blood vessels, thereby reducing the incidence of heart disease and hypertension.

Green Tea: It is full of **anti-aging vitamins**, lowers cholesterol, improves circulation and protects against skin cancer and arthritis. Green tea is an age old panacea. The Chinese discovered it thousands of years ago and found that it helped in warding off infections and it made you feel good and energetic.

Herbal Tea: It contains **rosemary, oregano, basil,** peppermint, and dash of turmeric. It also acts as antioxidant and has been found to be very useful in diabetes and arthritis.

Beta-carotene: It is also called pro-vitamin A. It is an important fat-soluble antioxidant. It also decreases the risk of increased blood clotting.

Minerals: These are iron, copper, zinc, selenium, magnesium and chromium that also act as antioxidants.

Zinc: It is found in seafood, legumes, nuts and dairy products. A diabetic requires about 30 mg per day.

Magnesium: It is found in nuts, wheat germ, seafood, broccoli and banana. An average of 300 mg is needed per day. Routine evaluation of serum magnesium levels is necessary as deficiency of this element can cause **insulin resistance**, carbohydrate intolerance and hypertension. A daily dosage of 30 mg is recommended.

Selenium: It is found in whole grain, dairy products, fish, mushrooms and nuts. About 200 microgram is needed per day.

Chromium: It is required for the optimum utilization of glucose and insulin. It is found in whole grain, broccoli, black pepper, oranges, grapes and cheese. A daily dosage of 300 mg is required. Administration of this element has shown improvement in both mild glucose intolerance and frank diabetes. It also improved lipid variables in type 2diabetes, in a study carried out in the Chinese population. Women with gestational diabetes were also seen to benefit with chromium intake. Recent research has shown that steroid therapy increases the loss of chromium and replacement of this mineral can reverse steroid induced diabetes.

Garlic and Onion: These have significant blood sugar lowering action, which is due to the sulphur containing compounds, e.g. **allylproply disulphide** present in onion and **diallyl disulphide oxide** present in garlic. Also, onion has a compound called **quercetin**, especially in the skin, which helps to decrease eye problems associated with diabetes.

Coenzyme Q10: It is vital in the utilization of oxygen by the cells, thereby being essential in the healthy sustenance of the cells. The secretion of this enzyme, like many others, slows down as age advances and body suffers from its deficiency. This compound is marketed as tablets and dose prescribed is 60 mg per day.

Soy Foods: Soy foods are obtained from soy beans. These are known as **cholesterol killer**. Soy foods have gained lot of popularity these days. The reason for this is the effect of soy on blood cholesterol. It has been found that when people with high cholesterol levels, replaced animal proteins in their diet by soy proteins, the levels of total cholesterol, triglycerides, and LDL cholesterol in the blood decreased while the level of HDL cholesterol increased. Scientists have noted that in countries like China and Japan where soy foods constitute part of the staple diet, the incidence of heart attack and osteoporosis is low. Also, the incidence of certain cancer, including breast cancer, ovarian cancer and cancer of prostate is much lower as compared to their incidence in America. Soybeans are legume and like other beans contain certain chemicals known as **isoflavones** or **phytoestrogens**. These chemicals especially one called **genistein**, is similar to **human estrogens**. These substances are weaker than human estrogens and when ingested, probably block the action of normal stronger estrogens present in the body by blocking the receptors. Despite research in this field, it is still not known what component in the soy protein is responsible for lowering blood cholesterol levels, or the mechanism by which it operates.

Soybeans: These are also a good source of calcium, copper, magnesium and many B vitamins. These are also a rich source of protein. These are also high in fiber content. Soy has low glycemic index of 18 only. It is widely believed that regular consumption of soy enhances body's ability to:

- Decrease fat storage
- Increase fat burning rate
- Increase lean muscle mass
- Provide energy for activity
- Lower blood cholesterol, risk of heart disease and stroke
- Minimize insulin fluctuations

Certain other food supplements are also recommended for diabetics.

Alfa Lipoic Acid: It is considered to be a powerful antioxidant. It improves the effectiveness of other antioxidants especially vitamins C and E. It may help in the utilization of insulin, reducing insulin resistance, thereby improving glucose utilization. It repairs nerve damage and help in the treatment of diabetic neuropathy. Visual improvement in patients of glaucoma is reported. Recommended daily intake is 100-800 mg. However, research in its utility is still continuing.

Vanadyl Sulphate: It is believed to help in proper metabolism of glucose. Patients should not take it with kidney insufficiency.

Aloe Vera: It is a wonder herb that has been in use for hundreds of years. Its benefits have been described in ancient Indian text. It contains many important ingredients including vitamins C and E, some essential minerals and amino acids. It also contains **saponins** and **lignins** that help to bind toxic waste in the body. It is a potent stimulant of immune system of the body and helps curb infections and heal wounds. It is also a powerful antioxidant. The plant extract has been used for the treatment of skin burns in ancient era. It is a herb with succulent juicy interior and thorny exterior. It is very bitter in taste. Some people eat it raw while others prefer it cooked.

Spices: These such as cinnamon, turmeric, cloves, coriander and cumin are believed to help potentiate the action of insulin.

Diet for Diabetics

A sensible diet is a **balanced diet** based on cereals as staple food, with lots of fruits and vegetables. One must go for a vegetarian rather than non-vegetarian diet, having whole fruit rather than fruit juice which is devoid of fibers, moderate amount of dairy products and plenty of plain water rather than colas and aerated soft drinks. It is also advisable to eat homemade meals rather than indulge in fast food. Consider replacing animal proteins by plant proteins, as animal food is devoid of fiber.

In ancient India, when Ayurveda was the mode of treatment, doctors prescribed apples to relieve diarrhea. Apples are rich in pectin, the soluble fiber. Fiber, as mentioned earlier regulates intestinal motility, reduces absorption of cholesterol, thereby decreasing risk of heart disease and cancer. Green leafy vegetables are a rich source of fiber and minerals. Carrots have beta-carotene with all its advantages. Cranberry juice helps to kill bacteria.

Cereals are the staple diet all over the world. While pasta is preferred in Italy, chapattis are preferred in India, bread in Britain and tortillas in Mexico. Each preparation is inspiring in its own right. Although, they vary in starch content, but all share low fat content and have fair amount of proteins. They are all tremendously satisfying. No meal is complete without cereals. While wheat remains the main source, other grains such as rice and oatmeal are equally good. The US Department of Agriculture food pyramid recommends that most people eat from six to eleven servings from the cereal, rice and pasta group.

It is recommended that one should not take more than two eggs per week, not more than 4 oz of cheese, not more than 4 oz of red meat, not more than 8 oz of poultry, and minimum of three fish meals per week.

It is advisable to take chicken without skin, as skin is rich in saturated fats. Another method to decrease fat content of poultry and red meat is to boil them before cooking and throw away the water. Never use this water for soups or anything else. Avoid rich creamy sauces in your meals. Take clear soups instead of creamy preparations. Take lot of salads as appetizers, rather than fried preparations.

An average 1800-2000 calories required by an adult diabetic male, would include the following per day.

1. Six helpings of cereals.
2. Three helpings of vegetables.
3. Three helpings of dairy products.
4. Two helpings of fruits.
5. Two helpings of meat or fish or poultry.

One helping of cereal = one piece of bread = one small ready to eat tortilla = half cup of cooked cereal or pasta or rice = puffed cereal = ½ cup cornmeal.

One helping of vegetable = one cup of leafy vegetables = two third cup of cooked vegetables.

One helping of fruit = a medium apple or banana or orange or half grape fruit.

One helping of dairy products = half cup of milk = half cup yogurt = half oz of cheese.

One helping of meat = 2 oz of cooked lean meat, fish or poultry = half cup of cooked beans = 2 tablespoons of peanut butter = one egg.

Table 15.3 Nutrient Composition per serving in grams

Foods	Protein	Fat	Carbohydrate	Fiber	Calories
Vegetable	3	0	11	1-3	50
Fruits	0	0	20	1-3	80
Breads	2	0	15	1-4	70
Legumes	7	0.5	15	6-7	90
Fats	0	5	0	0	45
Milk*	8	0	12	0	80
Meats	7	3	0	0	55

* This means that 1/2 cup of low fat milk = 1 serving, has negligible fat, 8 gms protein, 12 gms carbohydrate and yields 80 calories.

Exercise

Exercise is a key area in the management of diabetes. There are many advantages of active exercise. For one, it helps to burn down calories, and it has been found that half an hour of moderate exercise brings the blood glucose level down by nearly 40 mg %.

The increased metabolic rate induced by activity, continues to remain high for quite sometime even after the cessation of activity. The most beneficial effect is the improvement of circulation to every organ of the body. This improved blood supply provides adequate nutrition to the cells, and removes waste material. Most important is the improved oxygen supply to the tissues, which helps them to better utilize food and improve their vitality and well being. Exercise increases the muscle mass of the body, which raises the metabolic rate. It also increases the strength of the heart and the circulation in the blood vessels of the heart, improves the stroke volume, thereby decreasing the incidence of angina and heart attack.

Exercise burns down calories and helps to reduce obesity, thereby the severity of diabetes is reduced and in many patients, the dose of insulin and other anti-diabetic drugs are significantly reduced. Sedentary lifestyle has been linked to 28% of deaths from leading chronic diseases.

Some of the important benefits of exercises are listed below:

- Exercise should be encouraged not only because of its beneficial effects on **blood pressure, cardiovascular conditions, diabetes** and **osteoporosis**, but also because it improves the mood and cures insomnia.
- It is believed that **improved circulation to the brain** helps to secrete certain hormones which elevate the mood of the person, helps him perform better, gives him a sense of satisfaction, eliminates worries and induces sound sleep. It is well known that a laborer sleeps much better than an executive.
- Exercise raises the level of HDL cholesterol and decreases the risk of coronary heart disease, produces sustained lowering of both systolic and diastolic blood pressures and also decreases the risk of cancer.
- Many a time, there is some excuse or the other, which prevents us from a daily workout. Either our life is a hectic swirl, or we are too tired, or there is no proper health club accessible to us, or something else. None of these reasons should deter us. The greatest motivation for exercise is the knowledge that exercise helps us to keep **agile and healthy**. All that is required, to feel fit and healthy, is to incorporate little more physical activity in our daily routine.
- Even when there is no health club available to us and life is very busy, there is always time for a stroll in the lawn or a leisurely walk on a footpath or in a mall. It is not necessary to have high intensity workouts, especially if one is old and somewhat disabled. A 30 minute daily walk has significant health benefits. It decreases blood pressure, decreases blood cholesterol, improves heart function and reduces risk of heart disease.
- **"Strenuous aerobic exercise is great if you are in decent shape and enjoy it,"** explains **Dr. Duncan** of the Cooper Institute for Aerobics Research in Dallas, But it is not necessary. What counts is, exercise regularly. If you become a little more active in your daily life and stick with it, your health improves significantly.

Dr. James Rippe, M.D., director of the Exercise Physiology and Nutrition Laboratory at the University of Massachusetts Medical Center in Worcester, asked volunteers to walk on a treadmill at slow, medium and fast speed. "No matter at what speed they walked," Dr. Rippe explains, "everyone felt equally less tense and stressed afterward."

Before you start any exercise program, it is advisable to have complete physical examination by your physician, especially in men above the age of 40 and in women above 50. Your limitations or disability, if any, must be taken into consideration before you embark on any exercise schedule. There are different types of exercises- Yogic exercises aerobic and anaerobic.

Yoga or Yogic Exercises

"Yoga is fusion of science with philosophy." Yogic exercises are mild, performed very gradually without any jerks or violent movements. These exercises are designed to improve the **microcirculation** of the **tissues**, which is essential for the vitality of organs. Yogic postures or asanas cleanse the body and the soul alike. By improving microcirculation the toxins from the body are removed.

Yoga means union. The yogic postures are believed to unite the body to the mind. This sounds obscure. But a deep fundamental truth is hidden in this obscure message i.e., the truth of **supremacy of mind over body**, controlling its functions and channelizing its energies into productive activity. Yogic exercises allow the release of **positive neurotransmitters in the brain** that induce healthy activity in the body.

It improves flexibility of joints, increases strength of muscles, relieves mental stress; remove negative thoughts, stills the mind, and enables one to experience perfect relaxation and supreme tranquility. The key elements in yoga are proper breathing, gentle and proper exercises and meditation. **Meditation heals all ailments**.

Breathing Exercises

Breathing exercises are the most important. These exercises improve the total breathing capacity of the lungs, eliminate toxins and improve the oxygen saturation of the blood, and increases oxygen delivery to the tissues. This is vital for burning down glucose to obtain energy. Lack of oxygen to the tissues depletes them of energy and cause fatigue. Yoga lays stress on exhalation rather than inhalation and it teaches to breathe through the nose. Some of the easy and important asanas are detailed below. In between the asanas and also at the beginning and end of yogic exercises it is important to perform the corpse pose. All asanas are to be performed on the floor. The person should be completely at ease and the environment should be absolutely peaceful. Best time to do yoga is early in the morning. It may be done late in the evening, but whatever the time there should be no rush or hurry.

Corpse Position

Lie on the back and keep the arms at the sides, at an angle of about 45 degrees. The palms should face upwards, the legs straight and feet in relaxed position and about 20 inches apart. Close the eyes and relax all muscles in the body. Stay in this position for few minutes and experience the total relaxation of the whole body.

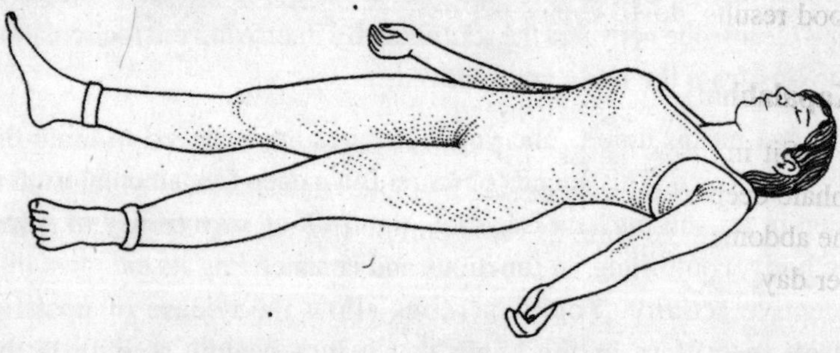

Abdominal Breathing

Lie flat on the back, placing one hand on your abdomen and the other arm by the side. Inhale deeply, while you feel the abdomen rising and then exhale while you feel the abdomen falling. This exercise enables the air to enter the lowermost part of the lungs and exercises the diaphragm.

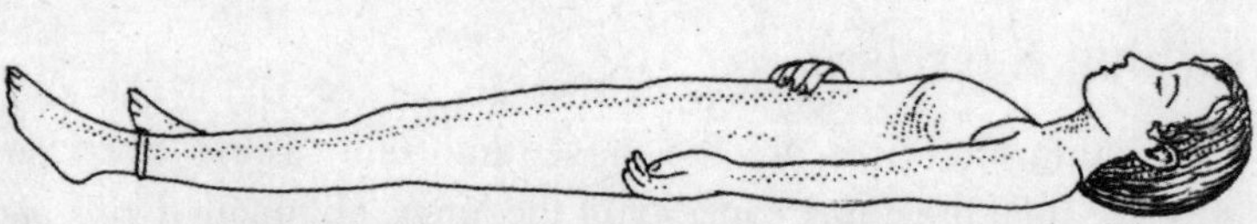

Alternate Nostril Breathing

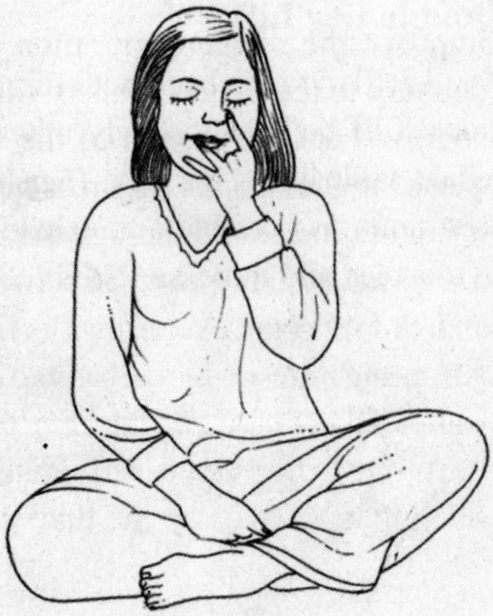

Sit in a comfortable cross-legged position with the spine and neck held straight. Hold the head erect and close the eyes. Put left hand on the left knee. Use right hand to close and open each nostril alternately. Hold the right hand in Vishnu Mudra position, which means keeping the thumb, little finger and ring finger extended and folding the remaining two fingers into the palm. Next close right nostril with the thumb and inhale through the left nostril to a count of four. Then close both nostrils with thumb and extended fingers to a count of 16. Next release the thumb and exhale through the right nostril to a count of 8. Repeat the three steps closing the left nostril instead of the right in the first step. These six steps form one cycle. For good results, do 10 cycles per day.

Kapalabhati

Sit in crossed-legged position keeping both hands on the knees. Inhale deeply and then exhale by rapid contractions of the muscles of the abdomen. Perform 25 rapid pumping in each cycle and do 3 cycles per day.

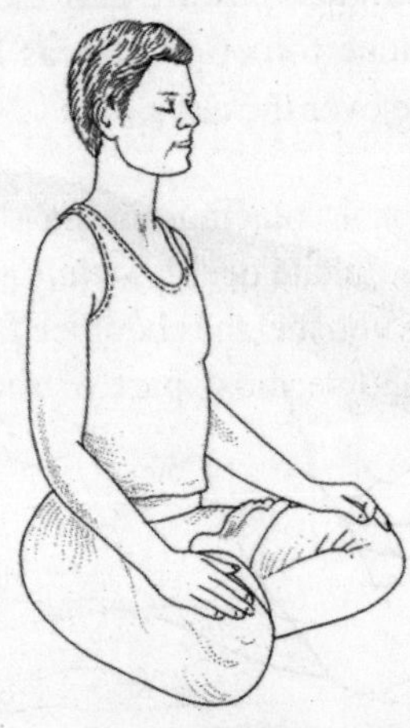

Double Leg Lift

Lie flat on the back with feet together and keep both hands by the sides. Lift both legs slowly upwards keeping the knees straight and inhale while lifting the legs. Then lower the legs slowly keeping the legs as straight as possible and exhale while lowering the legs. Start with five cycles and increase to ten.

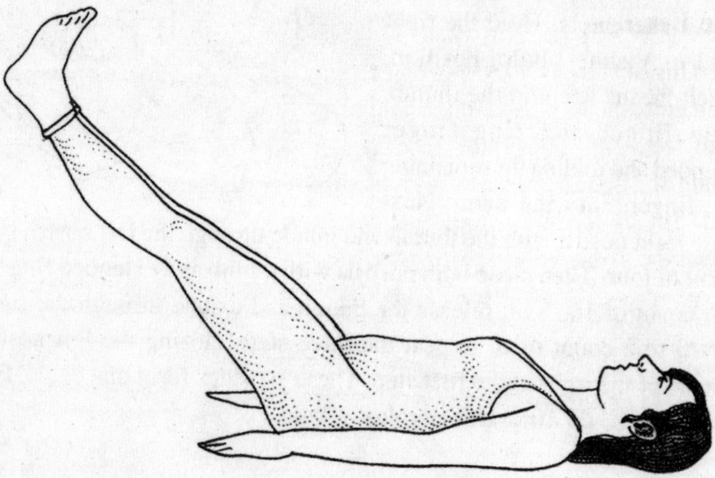

Forward Bend

This posture helps to strengthen the muscles of the spine and the abdomen. More important it improve the vitality of the organs of the abdomen. It is head to knee posture and the touching of forehead to knees should not be done forcefully. Do as much as is possible. You will gradually improve over the days.

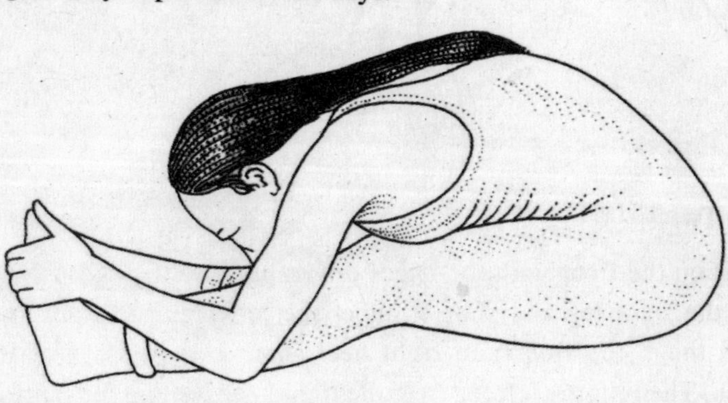

To begin with, sit with your legs straight in front of you. Keep your spine straight and while inhaling take your arms up parallel to your head. While exhaling, bend forward at your hips, hold the big toe between thumb and index finger and try to bring your forehead to touch the knees. Hold for 30 seconds and then stretch up. Repeat three times.

Side Bend

This posture is good for diabetes as well as for lower back pain. Stand erect on your feet. Inhale and jump your feet apart about two and a half feet. Turn your right thigh, leg and foot 90 degrees to the right. Exhale and bend your trunk to right, gripping right ankle with the right hand. Stretch the left arm in line with the shoulder. Turn and look up. Repeat the same with the left side.

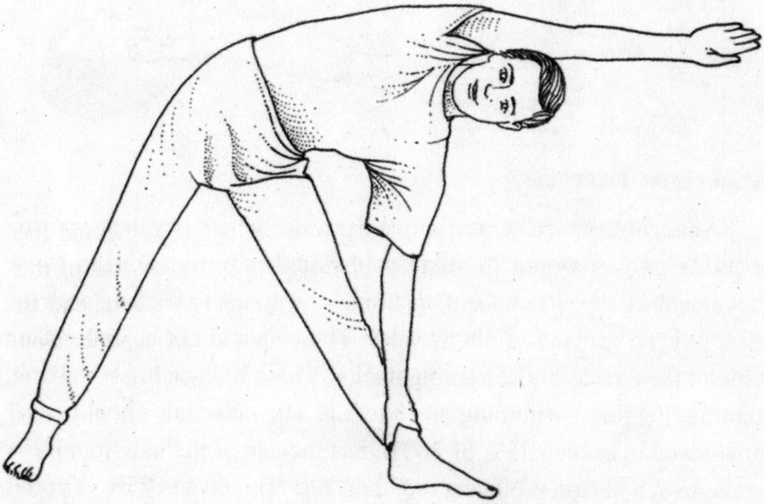

Spine Twist

Sit on the floor with the knees drawn close to the chest. Next, lower the right leg and slide it under the left leg. The right knee should touch the floor and right heel should be in front of left buttock. Then lift the left leg over the right knee putting the left foot on the outside of the right knee. Straighten the back and turn to the left putting the left hand behind the right foot. Bring the right arm over the left leg and place the right hand in front of right foot. Repeat the steps on the other side. This forms one cycle. Start with one cycle and increase to three.

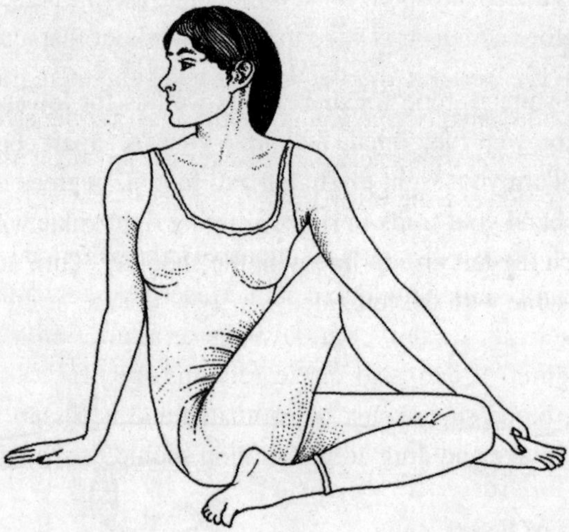

Anaerobic Exercise

Anaerobic exercises are active exercises where physical exertion requires extra oxygen to sustain physical activity. During these movements, the heart rate and breathing rate go up, to keep up with the extra oxygen demand of the muscles. These should not be undertaken without the advice of the treating doctor. These include brisk walking, running, jogging, swimming and cycling. The pulse rate should never be allowed to exceed 75% of 220 minus the age of the individual. For example, if a person is 60 year oid, then 220-60=160 and 75% of 160 is 120; hence the pulse rate should not exceed 120. In these activities, the energy needed is derived from the anaerobic metabolic pathway resulting in the formation of lactic acid, which accumulates in the muscles. As activity ceases, the negative balance of oxygen is restored and lactic acid is metabolized.

Aerobic exercises do not require extra load of oxygen and therefore do not put extra stress on heart and lungs. These include static cycling, workout on **treadmill**, weight lifting and similar exercises in the gymnasium.

The question that now arises is how much exercise is required? How hard one must work and for how long? The best person to monitor this is the person himself. Heart rate and fatigue levels are easy parameters to depend upon. What is moderate for one person may prove strenuous for another. It is wise to do the workout that agrees with the individual. It is better to start at a lower level and then gradually build up. As the body adapts, one can gradually increase the effort. Only the individual can determine how hard an exercise to start with and the rate at which to increase the effort.

These exercises need not be intensive to be beneficial. In diabetics, exercise can produce hypoglycemia. Hence, it is essential to have a snack, such as a candy bar, always available to you. Besides hypoglycemia, it can also cause rebound hyperglycemia. In such situations, blood sugar must be estimated and necessary adjustments with food intake and drug administration should be made.

Duration of Exercise

The total duration of exercise recommended per day is about an hour.

- Of this moderate exercise should be done for more than half an hour.
- Vigorous exertion should not exceed 20 minutes. The exercise should be build up gradually. Walking is one of the best forms of exercise, especially when undertaken early in the morning. Brisk walking sets up blood-pumping action in the calf muscles of the leg and is considered as one of the best forms of exercising the heart. Bones stay fit and maintain their strength and density by working against gravity. Jogging and squash are now considered to be the worst forms of strenuous exercise as the speed of blood circulation increases and this speeds up arteriosclerosis in the vessels.

Advantages of Exercise

To sum up exercise has the following benefits :

1. It increases muscle strength, stamina and flexibility.
2. It increases power of heart muscle.
3. The metabolic rate remains high even after the cessation of activity.
4. It helps control body weight.
5. It lowers blood sugar.
6. It lowers blood pressure.
7. It improves body circulation.
8. It increases HDL cholesterol levels in the blood.
9. It decreases stress and anxiety and elevate mood.
10. It increases sensitivity to insulin.
11. It improves sleep and minimize insomnia.
12. It reduces risk of heart attack and stroke.
13. It boosts the immune system and improves resistance to infections.

Table 15.4 Calories Burned in Different types of Exercise in an Adult, of an Average of 150 lbs Weight.

Activity for Half-Hour	Calories Burned
Brisk walking	160
Running	350
Swimming	130
Tennis	180
Football	220
Dancing, golf, baseball	130
Sleeping	30
Gardening	100
Yoga	100
Table work	60
Standing	40

Planning Exercise

While planning exercise few points must be kept in mind.

1. The type of exercise that can be done on daily basis.

2. The type of exercise that is safe, keeping in mind the status of the heart and the blood pressure.
3. The type of exercise, which will not affect any of your disability, which you might have, in an adverse manner.

For example, it is not safe for a person with arthritis of knee joints to workout on a treadmill, as this will further injure the joints. Static cycling is advisable in such situations.

Chapter 16

OBESITY

"Environment exposes what we inherit."

Obesity is now a global issue. It is of worldwide concern and there is need to tackle it on war footing. How to tackle obesity? It is a million dollar question. The causes and management of obesity is discussed in the following pages. Mechanisms that control hunger and appetite as well as the role of leptin are mentioned.

Long back, one day I asked my maidservant, named Akhtri, a poor widow with four kids to rear, "Why is it so difficult to loose weight? She retorted back, "Have you seen any poor person obese or overweight?" That was a hard-hitting truth. The poor people do lot of physical labor to earn their livelihood and eat only bare minimum to survive. They cannot afford the luxury of indulgence.

Obesity is central to the theme of diabetes, especially in NIDDM and IGT. Management of obesity is vital to the health of one and all. Reduction of weight is easier said than done. Obese people are 40 times more likely to develop diabetes than non-obese people. Obesity is one of the most common disorders and among the most frustrating and difficult to manage. Needless to mention, eating and exercise are the two ultimate factors that determine weight.

Management of Obesity

Although, sedentary lifestyles and overeating are the two main factors, there is evidence that genetic factors also influence development of obesity.

Many aspects of eating need to be dealt with. When to eat, how to eat, what to eat and how much to eat is critical. To be able to do this in an intelligent and scientific manner, it is crucial to understand the biology of hunger.

Biology of Hunger

Hunger is a powerful biological drive designed by nature for human survival. How much you eat is not always a matter of willpower, so much is inborn and so much is environmental. Availability and display of delicious food is the trigger that stimulates the brain to turn on the desire to eat into the actual act of eating. Trying to override one's basic instinct for nutritional need by dieting can be counterproductive as this may trigger the mechanism that turns on the appetite.

Hunger is regulated by a complex system of chemicals that communicate with brain and other systems of the body. Signals are passed back and forth from the brain to other parts of the body. The stomach, the fat stores of the body, the levels of blood glucose and the endocrine glands play significant role in this complex network.

The brain is the **center stage**. It receives messages from different parts of the body; processes the information and then sends down instructions. There is a specific area in the brain, called the **hypothalamus**, which contains the appetite center that determines when to eat and how much to eat. When the blood glucose level in the blood falls or when glycogen stores in the liver are depleted, then body reacts.

Chemical Messengers to Control Hunger

A neurotransmitter NPY, a kind of chemical messenger is released from the hypothalamus, which spurs the desire to eat sweets and carbohydrates. When one skips breakfast, the secretion of NPY is increased and by lunch time one's system is set to have a carbohydrate binge. In order to avoid such situation, it is advisable not to skip one's breakfast. Stress and dieting are also said to increase NPY secretion.

Serotonin is another chemical neurotransmitter that comes into action when one is full and has eaten his share of carbohydrates. It acts as negative feedback and informs the brain to turn off the secretion of NPY. When the level of serotonin rises, the level of NPY falls, sending a signal to the brain that food intake has been enough.

Douglas Coleman, working in 1960's, felt that eating behavior is controlled by a factor in blood, which in turn is controlled by one or more genes. He refused to believe in the prevailing view that obesity is a behavior problem and staunchly stuck to his theory and continued to search for the satiety factor. In 1980, Jeffrey Friedman at Rockefeller University started searching for the elusive ob (obese) gene. Rudy Liebel, at the same university, had also been searching for Coleman's satiety factor and ob gene. Liebel like Coleman thought that satiety factor was produced by fat cells. Liebal had worked with experimental mice, with obese and diabetic patients and was obsessed with the idea that there was something amiss in obese persons-the missing link that tells the body to eat or not to eat. He felt certain that genetics played an important role in determining weight regulation in humans. The BMI of identical twins was remarkably similar even when they were raised in separate environment. The BMI of adopted children correlated with their biological parents and not with their adoptive parents. In 1986, Friedman and Liebal started their hunt for the ob gene and located 4 genes. In 1991, a protein molecule that had the making of Coleman's satiety factor, produced in fat cells and coded for by a mutant gene found in obese mice (ob mice), was discovered. The satiety protein coded by ob gene was named leptin after the Greek word lepto meaning slim. Stephen O'Rahilly at Cambridge University located a Punjabi family, which had migrated to London from India years earlier, with very obese parents and siblings. He found the family to be deficient in leptin production similar to the ob mice.

Leptin is a cytokine (protein molecule) secreted by the fat stores of the body. When fat stores are full, adequate amount of leptin is released. Leptin informs the brain to turn off the appetite mechanism. The reverse happens when fat stores are depleted. The release of leptin from fat stores is withdrawn and brain continues to send appetite signals. A gene controls the production of leptin.

Ob gene is a defective gene, which prevents the production of adequate amount of leptin. Those individuals who inherit this gene are unable to produce leptin even when their fat stores are full. Hence, they are unable to send signals to the brain to suppress appetite and continue to feel hungry and eat excessively. Humans with defective gene are also infertile.

Role of leptin Leptin is secreted by fat cells

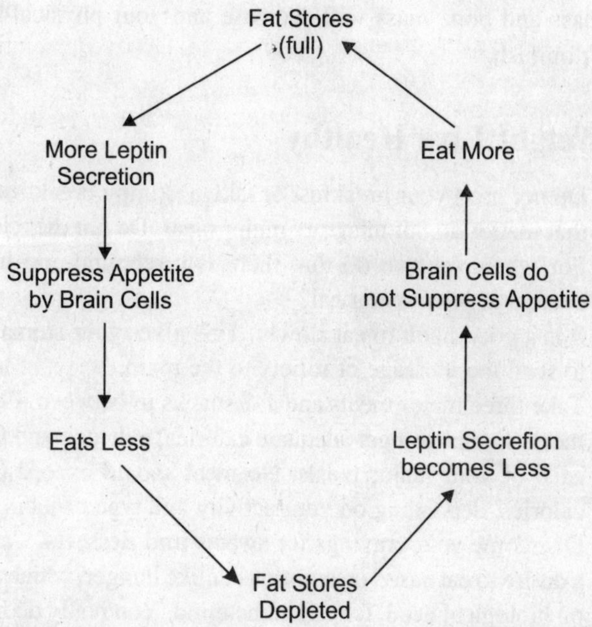

Fig. 16.1 Leptin acts on brain cells to suppress appetite. Withdrawal of leptin decreases appetite suppression.

Galanin is another transmitter, which is released when the fat stores are depleted and need to be replenished.

Cholecystokinin (CCK) is another chemical, which gets secreted when the stomach is full and there is feeling of satiety. This also acts on the brain inducing the brain to turn off the appetite mechanism. It takes the stomach about 20 minutes to get CCK into operation.

Obesity is difficult to treat, but there is no choice if one has to beat diabetes and other health problems linked with obesity. To do this, it is essential to inculcate certain healthy eating habits.

Mental Attitude

You have to decide in your mind what your goal is? You have to preserve yourself and keep going no matter what it takes. You will not achieve your goal in a few days; it may take many months. Remember there will be no miracles. Also remember that as you grow older, your muscle mass and bone mass will decrease and your physical activity may also diminish.

Lose Weight Live Healthy

1. Do not miss your breakfast or take a skimpy breakfast, or for that matter do not miss any major meal. Do not diet or starve. For whenever you do that there is a rebound and you will overeat at your next meal?
2. It is a good habit to eat slowly. This gives your stomach time to send the message of satiety to the brain.
3. Take three major meals and 1-2 snacks in between. Plan your meals so that you get adequate calories, nutrition and fibers in each of your major meals. No meal should exceed 600-800 calories, depending on your activity and type of job.
4. Overcome your cravings for **sweets and desserts**. Craving is a desire to eat based on emotions unlike hunger, which is based on biological need. It is all in the mind. You really do not need these extra calories, which will only add to your weight and not provide any nutrition.
5. As a snack, take tea or coffee. This also helps to ward off the hunger pangs. An apple, taken, as a snack is a very good habit.
6. Always take small helpings and never take a second helping. Never overeat, for if you do that you set your stomach at a much higher level of satiety. The result of this is that you develop a tendency to eat more to get the feeling of satisfaction and fullness.
7. Eat more fruits and vegetables and avoid fatty foods, especially those that are rich in saturated fats.
8. Drink plenty of water and avoid soft drinks and alcoholic beverages.
9. For the obese, overeating as a result of emotional reactivity can be a problem. A study conducted by **Micheal Lowe** of Rutgers University and **Edwin, Jr.**, of Washington University, showed that obese women were more emotionally reactive and more likely to engage in emotional eating as compared to those with normal weight.

10. Anger, stress or loneliness can be an emotional factor, tempting one to indulge in eating. Overcome this habit by engaging in some constructive activity such as going out for a walk or to a gym for a workout.

To sum it all, losing weight and keeping it off is not easy at all. But losing weight has so many health benefits and makes you feel so much smarter and better that it should become the first priority in your life.

Research shows that many people underestimate how much they eat and wonder why they don't lose weight on their "diets". Actually, the problem is people do not keep track of the calories they consume and often indulge in delicious fatty meals. Eat less means eat less calories and the easiest way is, to cut out saturated fats in your diet. Fats are the most concentrated source of calories and the least beneficial form of food. Make it your mission to succeed; adopt healthy eating habits and remain active.

Chapter 17

MANAGEMENT OF STRESS

"Knowledge is power no doubt. Know yourself first."

Stress is an elusive phenomenon. At times, circumstances are such that stress becomes inevitable. Harmful effects of stress are mentioned. The following paragraphs discuss the generation of stress and how to negate it.

Stress is one of the most important contributing factors to any disease. Management of any disease is incomplete without management of stress. Stress is in the mind, and in order to deal with stress we must analyze it from all angles and all aspects that impinge on the mind. We must understand the genesis of stress, the way in which it affects the body mechanisms and the best we can do to cope with it.

The phenomena of stress are most elusive to define. Perhaps, the only phase in man's life that is free from stress, is during infancy and early childhood when the mind is void of hate, jealousy and ego. As the human mind develops and grasps the complexity of the society around him, he becomes conscious of himself and aware of his needs and desires, he experience stress. Stress management is perhaps the most difficult aspect to be dealt with. It is one of the most important single environmental factors that precipitate a disease in a genetically predisposed individual. Stress causes the release of certain hormones from the brain which suppress the immune system, making the body susceptible to disease.

Excessive Desires–the Root Cause of Stress

Perhaps the root cause of stress in life is desire. There is desire to possess wealth, desire for power and promotion and desire to love and to be loved. The response to stress depends on each person's individuality and personality. Desire is like a **spider's web** that entangles and devours. There is a continuous entanglement in the web of desire and want, and the more one tries to get out of it the more entangled one gets, as one advances in life. One gets entangled more and more and there is a constant fear of getting devoured by the spider.

In this world of cut throat competition and rivalry, one often suffers from **inflated ego**. When one views the life in its entire perspective, one realizes how absurd all this is and how foolish it is to burden the mind with such afflictions. It is wiser to free the mind of such shackles that cause so much distress and agony.

How Does One Deal with Stress?

Can we free ourselves of all our desires and ambitions? If we can do that, then one wonders what this life is meant to be. As long as we live we cannot escape these situations and we have to learn to cope with adversities and learn to adjust and deal with the situation. **Alcohol and drugs are no answer to ones problem**. Such recourse only exposes our weakness. Anger, fear and anxiety are mere expressions of our inability to deal with the stressful situations.

Perhaps the answer to this lies within ourselves. We have to work out a solution ourselves. It must be positive and constructive. There is evidence that the way we feel and think has a tremendous effect on our body functions. The level of optimism and the degree of our positive mental attitude determines, to a large extent our well-being. Those with positive attitude and optimism view their misfortune as temporary setbacks and move forward in life.

The first step towards this goal is to take personal responsibility for one's mental attitude and not bear grudge towards others. Once we take an inward journey, passions slowly ease. At this juncture, we make our commitment towards our health and our goal. The path chosen has to be a middle path and certainly the path we have the faith to tread on. We have to find the strength within ourselves to meet the situation.

We derive this strength from our faith in God, for faith in God is faith in ourselves.

Influence of Prayer on Stress

We derive this internal strength by praying to God. Prayer is a great panacea of many maladies. We can pray to God in following ways:

1. One of the ways of prayer is to love and respect all Gods creations, especially our fellow beings.
2. Another form of prayer is right karma or deeds.
3. Pray by reading *Gita, Bible* or *Quran*. Reading Holy Scriptures and chanting hymns eases stress. The abstractions of Upanishads are worthy attractions.

Benefits of Prayer

The psychological and spiritual benefits of faith and prayer are tremendous. The body heals and tranquility settles in. When we pray, a fleet of thoughts stream through our mind. These thoughts create positivism that impinges on the border of yogic realm. The chanting of OM, a mantra induces a state of mind that experiences a total and sublime happiness that only comes with total detachment from all earthly materialism. This is what is known as **nirvana** in **Vedic** terms.

At times I pray, O God, take me into that realm of tranquility where the shackles of materialism do not stifle the soul, where the clarity of thought is not shrouded by hatred and jealousy, where realization is not made blunt by such complexes as inferiority or superiority. At this moment, I am reminded of a verse written by the Noble Laureate **Rabindranath Tagore** - "O God, wake my countrymen into that morning where the mind is free and the head is held high."

While we live in this world, we cannot be totally detached. The great Indian philosopher and founder of Buddhism, Gautam Buddha, ordained a different philosophy wherein he advocated a middle path. Here one is not unduly attached to materialism for it to become an ailment, nor is one completely detached so as not to fulfill ones obligations to the mother earth to whom one owes ones existence. This is perhaps a more practical approach.

Effect of Meditation on Stress

Meditation is one of the ways, which enables us to relieve ourselves of stress. It helps us to seek and find God. Prayer and good living are also paths that lead to enlightment and to his kingdom. Prayer, especially in deep concentration, bans disruptive and negative thoughts from the mind. Yoga helps to achieve the same objective. It stills the minds and calms the soul.

Meditation has been proved to decrease the secretion of cortisone into blood. **Cortisone** is a hormone released during stress and it reduces immunity, raises blood pressure and damages the tissues. Another hormone released by the body during stress is **adrenaline** secreted by the adrenal glands. This chemical constricts the blood vessels, reduces the supply of oxygen and nutrients to the tissues and compromises vitality of the tissues. A sustained situation of such a state predisposes to hypertension or high blood pressure.

Transcendental meditation is another technique in which repetition of a mantra such as OM is used to focus the mind. Similarly, an object or picture can be used to focus or concentrate the mind. In the beginning, meditation needs to be practiced for 20 minutes, twice a day. Later, the time can be reduced when the person becomes more proficient and he can achieve the same benefit in shorter period of time.

Other Methods to Relieve Stress

There are several other methods to relieve stress besides prayer and meditation. Simple procedures like **deep breathing**. Massage of neck and shoulder muscles, listening to good music, smelling perfumes as lavender also to help relieve tension and stress.

Lying in a hot water tub or spa for 15-30 minutes goes a long way in alleviating stress. This endeavor relaxes the muscles, improves the circulation, relieves stiffness of the joints, opens up the skin pores, makes the person feel good and put a stop to a hectic regime.

When sadness clouds happiness, watch a movie, which has comedy in it, or read some jokes that make you laugh. As an age old saying goes, **"Laughter is the best medicine."** When one is under stress, one tends to fall a prey to reactive eating. This habit should be overcome. Overeating must be avoided at all cost. Desire of eating is a weakness, which must be overcome. We must eat to live and not live to eat.

Chapter 18

MEDICATION

Medication should be the last resort. But if the doctor prescribes it, do not avoid it. The various allopathic medicines including oral drugs, insulin injections and combination therapy are discussed in detail in the following paragraphs. The mode of action of drugs and their side effects are mentioned.

Medication includes allopathic and ayurvedic drugs. No form of medication should be undertaken without the consultation of medical professionals. Certain herbs, which have been found to help regulate blood sugar levels, can be tried as adjuvant to conventional therapy.

When diet regulation, weight reduction and exercise do not help in controlling diabetes, emphasis is laid on allopathic medicines. Among the anti-diabetic drugs are oral tablets and insulin injections.

Oral Pills

First line of therapy is an oral pill. It is much easier to swallow a pill than take a shot. Moreover, it is easier to control diabetes with pills than insulin injection. It is recommended that therapy should always be instituted with lower dose and gradually increased till optimum control is achieved. Also, when mono-therapy fails **multiple drug therapy** is tried, either tablets with injection, or different class of pills. There are four main groups among the oral medicines given in the treatment of NIDDM or type 2diabetes.

1. The first group includes **sulphonylureas**, which act on the pancreas and increase the production of insulin.
2. The second group consists of **biguanides**, which act on peripheral tissues to lower blood glucose level, especially liver and decreases entry of glucose from liver into blood.

3. The third group is **A-glucosidase** inhibitors which decrease the absorption of glucose from intestine into blood.
4. The fourth group includes **thiazolidinediones**, which increase the entry of glucose from blood into peripheral tissues.

Sulphonylureas

Sulphonylureas are potent, and effective with relatively few side effects, but can cause weight gain and hypoglycemia. Also, after prolonged use, these may lose their effectiveness. This group of drugs is not used in type1diabetes. There is hardly any pancreatic tissue capable of producing insulin in type1diabetes. Hence, sulphonylureas, which have very little potentiating effect on the action of insulin on peripheral tissues and depend on functioning pancreatic tissue for their activity, have no significant role to play in these patients.

Sulphonylureas are most useful in nonobese type 2diabetes. In type 2 obese diabetes, control of the disease is first attempted by weight reduction, diet regulation and exercise. However, if these measures fail, then oral drugs are given. These drugs are also given in severe cases of type 2 obese diabetes. Sulphonylureas are contraindicated in patients with liver and kidney failure.

There are two generations of these drugs. The first generation compounds are used only in selected elderly patients with cardiovascular impairment. This group is less potent and less likely to produce hypoglycemia, which can prove very dangerous in elderly patients with compromised cardiovascular function and can precipitate heart attack.

Diabetic patients, who have failed to respond to the maximum dose of the most potent of first generation drugs, are given the second-generation drugs. These latter drugs are much more potent as compared to the first generation compounds and are more favored in younger adults. The second-generation drugs include **glyburide** (Diabeta, Micronase, Glynase), **glipizide** (Glucotrol) and **glimepiride** (Amaryl). Amaryl besides acting on the pancreas also increases the sensitivity of the peripheral tissues to the action of insulin. Amaryl is one of the **preferred drugs** and is often given in conjunction with insulin. This drug is not advocated in patients with ketosis and is not given in persons allergic to it.

Biguanides

This class of antidiabetic drugs used in type 2diabetes was introduced in 1950s. Phenformin was the first compound in this series. However, it was soon discontinued because of its association with lactic acidosis. Research led to the development of better products. The latest compound to be marketed is **metformin**.

Metformin, also called **glucophage**, is considered a safe drug and is now often used as first line of therapy in the treatment of NIDDM. It does not act on the pancreas to stimulate insulin release but acts on the peripheral tissue in bringing down fasting and postprandial blood sugar levels. It acts on the liver, preventing the formation and release of glucose from liver into the blood. It also helps in increasing the uptake of glucose from the blood, by the skeletal muscles. It is also believed to decrease glucose absorption from the intestinal tract. In some studies, it has been shown to decrease blood lipid levels. It has synergistic action with **glitazones** in lowering blood glucose levels. This drug causes the patients to lose weight. It is contraindicated in patients with hepatic and renal problems. It should not be given in persons taking alcohol.

The minor side effects reported are gastrointestinal symptoms such as nausea and vomiting. These effects are transient, dose related and are present at the initiation of therapy. It is a good drug given as adjuvant to diet alone or in combination with other oral tablets or insulin. It is administered in divided doses.

Alpha-Glucosidase Inhibitors

This group has two products, **acarbose** (precose) and **miglitol** (glyset). These drugs lower blood glucose levels by delaying the absorption of sugar in the intestinal tract. They have major effect on postprandial glucose levels, keeping the levels low and thereby also keep glycosylated hemoglobin low. These are not given in patients taking lispro (Humalog) insulin and contraindicated in patients with hepatic or renal impairment. These have mild side effects such as flatulence and diarrhea.

Thiazolidinediones

These include **glitazones, troglitazone** (rezulin) and **pioglitazone**.

Due to its effect on liver causing liver failure, rezulin has been discontinued. Two other products, related to rezulin and belonging to this category of compounds are available in the market. These drugs are considered safe and are gaining favour with doctors and patients. These are **actos** and **avandia**.

Actos

This drug is available in the form of tablets and is taken only once a day. It can be taken with or without meals, any time during the day. It helps to lower blood sugar levels. The most important feature of this preparation is, that it helps to sensitize tissues of the body to utilize better the insulin already present in the body. Insulin may be endogenous, which the body is making or exogenous, which the patients takes it in the form of injections. Actos works by treating **insulin resistance**, which is an important underlying defect present in type 2diabetes. It helps the body to use insulin more effectively and respond better to the insulin already available. Unlike the sulfonylureas it does not act by increasing insulin production by the pancreas. It may take few weeks before the effect of actos becomes manifest. Actos can be combined with the other antidiabetic drugs such as **insulin, metformin**, and **sulfonylureas**. Actos is also metabolized in the liver, which means it is broken down in the liver and excreted by the kidneys. Hence, it is mandatory to run tests for liver and kidney functions and to be sure that liver and kidney functions are normal before starting this drug.

Actos is contraindicated in type 1diabetes, pregnancy, lactation, ketoacidosis, congestive heart failure, edema or swelling of feet, liver or kidney disease and allergy to actos.

Actos is generally well tolerated by patients on clinical trials. However, patients have reported few side effects. These include upper respiratory tract infections, sore throat, sinusitis, headache and tooth disorder. Weight may increase with the use of this drug.

Other drugs are also available in the market. These include.

Repaglinide

It acts on beta cells in the pancreas and enhance the secretion of insulin. It is as effective as sulphonlyureas and prevents postprandial hyperglycemia.

D-phenylalanine Derivatives

They act on pancreas and stimulate rapid secretion of insulin. It helps to control hyperglycemia and reduce the increase in blood glucose levels that occur after ingestion of meals. **Starlix** is one of the available brands.

Insulin

This medicine is given as injection. It is imperative in the treatment of type1diabetes in which the beta cells in the pancreas are non-functional and cannot produce insulin at all. It is also indicated in patients of non-obese type 2diabetes where hyperglycemia fails to respond to diet therapy either alone or in combination with oral anti-diabetic drugs.

Insulin is also administered during pregnancy in diabetic women. A diabetic patient undergoing surgical intervention also needs to be put on insulin. Insulin preparations available in the market differ with respect to the animal species from which they are obtained, the degree of purity and solubility, and the time of onset and duration of action. Insulin preparations obtained from animal species other than human beings have the disadvantage of causing allergic reactions, as these preparations are foreign proteins. With the availability of highly purified human insulin, the complications associated with insulin injection have reduced considerably. The incidence of insulin allergy, the immune insulin resistance and lipotrophy at the site of injection has decreased. Human insulin is currently prepared by **recombinant DNA techniques**, which is a biosynthetic method. Commercial insulin preparations now available in the market are mainly of four types.

Regular ® insulin: It is short acting insulin. When given as subcutaneous injection, the action starts within 0.5-1 hr and lasts for 5-8 hours. It is clear crystalline preparation and its intravenous infusion is preferred in the treatment of acute diabetic complications, in perioperative period and in severe infections.

NPH insulin: It is intermediate-acting insulin whose onset of action is about 2-4 hours and the duration of action is about 18-24 hours. Lente insulin is also intermediate acting in nature.

Ultralente insulin: It is long-acting insulin. The action starts in

6-8 hours and lasts for 24-30 hours.

Lispro (Humalog) [H]: It is rapid acting insulin and must be given no more than 10-15 min before eating.

The new, Long-Acting Insulin, Glargine (Lantus): It has recently become available. It is taken once a day. This can be combined with short acting insulin for optimum control of diabetes.

It is customary to combine **short-acting insulin** with the **long acting insulin** to allow preprandial and postprandial daylong coverage by the drug. Stable premixed preparations containing different concentration of different types of insulin are available in the market. Insulin vials should be stored in refrigerator when not in use to avoid loss of bioactivity. They should not be stoned in freezer. A table given below shows the various insulin preparations available and in common use.

Table 18.1: Various Insulin Preparations in Common Use.

Human insulin	Onset of action	Peak of action	Duration of action
Rapid-Acting Lispro [H]	10-15 min	1-2 hrs	3-4 hrs
Short-Acting Regular [R]	0.5-1 hr	2-5 hrs	5-8 hrs
Intermediate-Acting NPH [N]	2-4 hrs	6-10 hrs	18-24 hrs
Intermediate-Acting Lente [L]	3-4 hrs	6-12 hrs	20-24 hrs
Long-Acting Ultralente [U]	6-8 hrs	Usually none	20-30 hrs

Site of Insulin Injection

The injection is given subcutaneously and any part of the body covered by loose skin can be used. It is recommended that the site of injection should be changed as injection at the same site results in **fibrosis** and **lipohypertrophy**, which delays insulin absorption from the site. It has been shown that regular insulin gets absorbed from the subcutaneous tissue of the abdomen most rapidly. It is therefore suggested that the abdominal site should be used to get better control of the disease. Methods of injection depend on the delivery system, which vary from simple syringe and needle to insulin pens and pumps.

Disposable plastic syringes with attached needles are available in 1 ml, 0.5 ml, and 0.3 ml sizes. In those cases, where low doses of insulin are prescribed it is convenient to use 0.5 ml or 0.3 ml size as that facilitates more accurate measurement of insulin taken. Disposable syringes can be reused till needles get blunt. The needles can be used 3-5 times without compromising on sterility, by covering the needle with the cap in between use.

Insulin pens are convenient devices that can be used in place of syringes and needles. These are useful in the hands of patients with poor eyesight or shaky hands. Reusable pens fitted with the cartridges are available and permit administration of accurate dose in a quick and easy way.

Chapter 19

HOME REMEDIES

Many years of experience and search has gone into the development and usage of these preparations. Most of the preparations are mild and have no side effects. However, no medication should be taken without professional consultation.

In ancient India, when the modern drug industry was non-existent, certain household remedies were in practice. These substances have been in use since time immemorial in the Indian subcontinent, having its inception in the Aryan period. As diet regulation continues to be an important and integral part of the management of diabetes, these remedies are derived from the common food items. Herbs and certain food ingredients that are helpful in diabetes are mentioned below.

Ginger

Ginger (Adrak) is the rhizome of the plant *Zingiber officinale*. It is used widely in India, as household remedy and forms one of the basic ingredients in Indian cookery. A preliminary research, carried out in alloxan induced diabetic rats and rabbits, has shown that administration of freshly extracted ginger juice had significant blood glucose lowering effect in these animals.

Indian Gooseberry

The Indian name is **amla** and the botanical name is *Emblica officinalis*. Amla is rich in Vitamin C. A tablespoonful of its juice mixed with a cup of bitter gourd juice taken daily is said to help stimulate the islets of Langerhans. Amla powder mixed with Jamun powder and bitter gourd powder are also very effective in the management of diabetes.

Jamun

This fruit is called **Jamun** in India, Java plum in English and the botanical name is *Syzgium cumini*. The whole fruit especially the seeds are considered very useful in tackling diabetes because of its stimulating effect on the pancreas. In Aryan time, even the bark of the Jamun tree was used in the treatment of diabetes.

Bitter Gourd or Plant Insulin

The Indian name is Karela and the botanical name is *Momordica charantia*. In India, gourd is considered specific in the management of diabetes. A group of British scientists has shown that bitter gourd has a compound with insulin like activity. It is called **plant insulin**.

Fenugreek

The Indian name is **methi** and the botanical name is *Trigonella foenum-graecum*. Fenugreek has got soluble fibers called mucilage and some other compounds, which help to lower blood sugar levels and raise HDL cholestrol. According to the Indian Council of Medical Research (ICMR), the fenugreek seeds are highly effective in the treatment of diabetes.

Lettuce, tomato and tender leaves of mango plant are considered useful and healthy constituents of the diet of the diabetic patients.

Black Gram

The Indian name is **masha/urad** and botanical name is Phaseolus roxburghi. It was used widely in ancient times for the prevention of complications of diabetes mellitus. Bengal gram, red kidney beans and mong (*Phaseolus munga*) are among the legumes most popularly advocated in diabetes. French beans (*Phaseolus vulgaris*) have been used in India since ancient times for the management of diabetes.

Guar

Cyamopsis psoralioides called **guar** in Hindi has been one of the most efficient and popular herb used in the management of diabetes. Its pod and seeds are used for treatment.

Curry Leaves

Murraya koenigi known as **curry leaves** are widely used in Indian culinary and is considered a good carminative and the infusion of leaves have blood glucose lowering effect.

Barley

Barley and its grasses are also considered good dietary constituents and are believed to boost the immune system and help to prevent diabetes, arthritis, heart disease and cancer.

Fruits

Grape seed extract is a useful dietary supplement as it is a strong antioxidant, It is said to prevent the breakdown of collagen, which is integral component of the body tissues. *Aegle marmelos* known as **bael** fruit in Hindi. The alcoholic extract of the roots and fruits of this plant have been shown to have hypoglycemic activity in albino rats. Banana is one of the most common fruits in tropical countries. The unripe banana is considered a good dietary constituent in diabetes.

Groundnut

Groundnuts are a rich source of niacin and useful in preventing the vascular complications of diabetes.

Holy Basil

Holy basil is also believed to lower blood glucose levels thereby helping diabetes.

All these household remedies were and are in common use in India. Recently, research in these food items has shown their utility.

Ancient Drugs used in Diabetes

Some simple drugs used in ancient times and still being used in Indian households are following.

Karavellaka (Sanskrit). The alkaloid extract of Momordia charantia. It produces hypoglycemia and hypocholesteremia. The effect starts in about 2 weeks time and becomes significant in three week onwards.

Madhunashini (Sanskrit) *Gymnema sylvestre*. Leaf extract of this plant helps to regulate glucose metabolism in diabetics.

Jambu (Sanskrit) *Eugenia jambolana*. This produces marked reduction of blood glucose levels and also brings down blood cholesterol.

Nimba (Sanskrit) *Azadirachta indica*. Hindi name is neem. The leaves are extremely useful in diabetes as they are potent hypoglycemic agents and reduce the clotting of blood thereby preventing vascular complications of diabetes.

Shilajitu: It has been widely used since ancient times as an antioxidant and is also known for its hypocholesteremic properties.

Yashada bhasma: It contains zinc, which helps in the metabolism of insulin.

Loha bhasma: It contains iron, which also helps in the metabolism of insulin.

Gugolipid

Gugolipid is a derivative of resin from the Commiphora mukul tree, and has been used in India since 600 BC. This has been used by Indians to treat lipid disorders and to alleviate the effects of overeating and overindulgence. This herb, which originated in north-central India, is found to decrease blood cholesterol levels. Dr. Szapary of the University of Pennsylvania, Philadelphia, who received a grant from NIH, has studied the effects of this herb in clinical trials. He reported that total cholesterol levels decreased by 12%, LDL by 13%, and triglycerides by 12%.

Gymnema Sylvestre

Gymnema Sylvestre (GS) belongs to the family of Asclepiadaceae. It is a wonderful medicinal plant found in India and Africa. Its distribution is now worldwide. Its utility as medicinal plant has been recognized in Japan and some other countries. In India, it has been used in Ayurvedic medicine for centuries and is popularly called Gurmar (gur in Hindi is sugar and mar means destroyer) due to its unique ability to blunt the desire for sweets. The leaf extract of GS has been used as a remedy for the diabetes in Indian traditional medicine. It is also believed to have antiviral, antiatherosclerotic, hypolipidaemic, and liver protective properties. It is also said to prevent **dental caries**. More recently, this plant has been picked up by natural products industry in North America and Europe. A number of herbal products containing extracts of GS are now available. Experimental studies in man and animals are being conducted to evaluate its effectiveness in lowering blood sugar levels. In vitro production of active ingredient in tissue culture is gaining worldwide popularity.

Gymnema extract is still being used in the management of diabetes in India in various combinations and formulations. It is believed to act in a manner similar to sulfonylureas. It is believed to act on the islets of Langerhans and **boost insulin secretion**. It also inhibits absorption of glucose from the intestinal tract into the blood. It also decreases the desire for sweets by blunting the sensation of sweet buds in the tongue. If the patient is on antidiabetic medication, the dose needs to be adjusted when adding gymnema to the drug regime.

There are many other drugs used in Ayurvedic branch of medicine but as there is no documented research on them, they are not being mentioned.

Chapter 20

Recent Advances in Diabetes

It is always rewarding to keep informed. Some of the recent research and discoveries are mentioned below.

Transplant Surgery

In 1921, Dr Paul Lacey of Washington University first reported that islet cell transplant could cure diabetes in experimental rats. *Dr David Sutherland* of the University of Minnesota proved that a patient, whose pancreas had been removed surgically, could achieve insulin independence by the re-transplantation of his or her islet cells.

Trials on Transplant Surgery

It has been a long and a lengthy endeavor to treat diabetes by transplanting beta islet cells of pancreas obtained from human cadaver into the patients of diabetes, especially in type 1 DM. Till now the attempts had **not proved** to be **very successful**. There are several factors, which have delayed the success of this technique. It is difficult to get healthy human islet cells and there is the problem of rejection of the transplanted tissue. Moreover, the patients have to be kept on strong immunosuppressive drugs, which have potentially dangerous side effects. Research is being carried out to overcome these hurdles.

In one experimental study, islet cells collected from rats were kept in a solution containing **alginate**. This treatment resulted in creating a hard shell around the cells with pores, which were large enough to allow the passage of insulin and glucose but small enough to prevent the entry of immune cells. These cells were then kept in the laboratory and were found to generate insulin and respond to changes in glucose levels in the environment. Human trials still remain to be conducted.

However, in May 2000, *Dr James Shapiroal* of the University of Alberta, Edmonton in Canada, reported success in islet cell transplant in eight patients suffering from type 1diabetes. These patients do not require insulin any more. However, these patients are kept on immunosuppressive drugs, so that their bodies do not reject the transplanted graft. These patients will have to be kept on these drugs indefinitely. The success in these cases has been attributed to new regime of immunosuppressive drugs. *Dr Thomas Starzl* of the University of Pittsburgh, a premier liver transplant researcher, pioneered the use of **FK 509**, an anti-rejection drug, used by the Edmonton group. Its long-term benefits await evaluation.

Although, these initial trials are encouraging it is still to be seen whether these procedures can be carried out in large population of patients. So far, the procedure has been done on very few patients and very little time has elapsed to know what unexpected complications and problems might crop up and how long the graft will survive.

Obstructions in Transplant Surgery

The biggest **hurdle in transplant surgery** is the availability of healthy human islet cell graft. A team at the University of California, San Diego, recently showed success in developing first human beta cell lines that secret insulin in response to glucose. This development may provide unconstrained source of beta cells for transplantation, overcoming the shortage of cells from organ donors. Further research will demonstrate whether these cells can be safely transplanted in patients with diabetes and whether these cells will retain the ability to produce insulin over the long periods of time. **Stem cell research** will open up new avenues of treatment and holds much promise.

Genetic Engineering Research in Transplant Surgery

A gene for **islet-neogenesis-associated protein** (INGAP) may help in changing the dormant cells in the pancreas into active insulin producing beta cells. This could benefit patients with both type 1 and type 2diabetes.

Gene mapping and gene therapy will open up new avenues in medicine. Research in this field will provide vast information and valuable clues in the functioning of individual genes. Long–term research in genetic engineering has the potential to develop insulin-secreting human cell lines and techniques of sustaining grafted cells by newer immunosuppressive methods and this could lead to new treatment approaches.

Doctors are now considering pancreatic transplant along with kidney transplant in cases of end stage renal disease where kidneys have failed and the only option left is **transplant surgery**. Since, patient has to undergo surgery anyway and live on immunosuppressive drugs, why not combine it with, pancreatic transplant also.

Insulin Therapy

Continuing research is coming up with new innovations in diabetes management. It is advisable to keep oneself abreast of the new developments. One of the most remarkable and recent research has been towards the development of an effective **insulin inhalation** delivery mechanism. This offers a major breakthrough in the management of diabetes. This is however, still in an experimental stage.

Many patients of diabetes depend on insulin injection for the control of their condition. Injections are painful, inconvenient and somewhat cumbersome. Aradigm Corporation is one of the companies working on developing inhalers for diabetes. These inhalers contain the medicine in aerosolized form. This mode of therapy is being used very frequently and successfully in the management of asthma. However, only a small fraction of the medicine present in the inhaler enters the airways, which makes this method of drug delivery rather expensive. Another difficulty encountered in the case of diabetes, is the delivery of the exact dose, which needs to be monitored precisely in cases of diabetes. The insulin used has been of the short-acting type. Efforts are being made to prepare aerosol molecules of longer acting insulin. Past research has shown that insulin can cross the fine membrane that separates the air sacs from the blood vessels in the lungs.

Leptin Injection

Obesity is a chronic disease rather than a behavioral disorder. It is a major predisposing factor in cardiovascular problems, diabetes and even in cancer. Maintenance of ideal weight is crucial to the prevention and management of diabetes. Hence, techniques to enhance weight loss may help in the prevention and treatment of diabetes. **Leptin is a hormone generated by the fat cells in the body and plays an important role in both food intake and regulation of body weight.** It is protein in nature. It acts on certain receptors in the brain, which in turn suppresses appetite, inhibits synthesis of fat in the fat cells and promotes burning of fat in the muscles of the body by increasing the metabolic rate. It is postulated that in obese individuals, the brain receptors do not respond to leptin adequately. Preliminary research has shown that synthetic form of leptin, when injected in obese individuals, helps in weight reduction. Several studies are in progress to study the effectiveness of leptin in weight reduction and glucose metabolism.

At the University of Texas, Southwestern Medical Center in Dallas, scientists injected recombinant adenovirus with leptin gene into healthy rats with normal body fat. The rats overproduced leptin, which resulted in the loss of body fat but no lean body mass. The insulin level in the animals dropped but there was no development of diabetes. It is believed that the animal's sensitivity to insulin is directly linked to fat stores in the body. **The more the fat in the body, the less is the sensitivity to insulin**. These findings may help in the understanding of insulin resistance in humans. In those individuals, who have insulin resistance; also have higher body mass index, percentage body fat, and amount of abdominal fat. It is possible that either the level of leptin is low or the brain receptors are resistant to leptin. **Johannsson**, in his research work, has shown that humans, who are obese and resistant to insulin, have higher concentration of leptin in their body, indicating thereby that brain receptors are resistant to leptin.

Regranex

Regranex (becaplermin) gel is a recent innovation in the field of biotechnology. It is a **cytokine** or **growth factor** derived from the platelets. Platelets are small cells present in the blood that help in its coagulation. Regranex has been shown to help in **healing of wounds** and **ulcers**. It promotes proliferation and migration of cells to the site of wound and helps in the synthesis of new tissues. It stimulates neovascularisation as well as the formation of connective tissues. The

FDA (Food and Drug Administration) has given its approval for this compound. It is a **topical ointment**, to be applied locally on wounds. It gets absorbed through the skin. It is a remarkable adjuvant in the treatment of diabetic foot ulcers. **Diabetic foot ulcers**, as is known, is a serious complication, which if untreated can result in **osteomyelitis** and even **amputation**.

AGEs

AGEs (advanced glycosylation endproducts) are compounds that are formed when blood glucose levels are high and glucose binds with proteins in blood and tissue fluids. It is a kind of **glue** that seals the pores in the blood vessels and interferes with the biological functions of body's cells. **AGEs** inhibitors are now available and are used to inhibit or slow the process of combination of glucose to proteins.

ARIs (aldose-reductase inhibitors) are compounds, which block the action of the enzyme, which causes accumulation of glucose by products. ARIs thus, prevent adherence of glucose by products to nerves and thereby protect the nerves. These two products are among the recent discoveries.

Memantin, another drug used in neuropathy, is under trial. **Tragretin** is a new compound, which has been found to decrease insulin resistance. However, it is still on clinical trial and not ready for use.

C-peptide

C-peptide is a substance normally produced by the body. It is a by-product of insulin synthesis. Its assay in blood helps to estimate the amount of insulin produced in the body. It has been found not only to prevent some complications of diabetes but also reverse them. Administration of C-peptide along with insulin in experimental rats reversed certain complications by nearly 70%.

Atorvastatin

Atorvastatin lowers plasma cholesterol by 32-38%, triglycerides by 15-25%, and LDL by 43-50%. Atorvastatin also lowers C-reactive protein and improves endothelial dependent vasodilation in type 2diabetes Endothelial cells form the inner lining of blood vessels. C-reactive proteins (CRP) are normally produced in the body and play significant role in inflammation.

Endothelial dysfunction is frequently found in diabetic subjects. Diabetic patients had higher levels of CRP than matched non-diabetic controls and both endothelial dependent and independent vasodilation was impaired. Atorvastatin treatment in type 2 diabetics not only decreased the levels of CRP but also significantly improved endothelial functions (The Journal of Clinical Endocrinology and Metabolism- Vol 87, No 2, 563-568).

New Drugs on Clinical Trial

Many new preparations are on clinical trials that will possibly treat and reverse the ravages of diabetes.

- **Byetta**, an injectable preparation, which mimics a naturally produced hormone that helps to control diabetes has been approved by FDA, USA. Byetta is given twice daily. A newer preparation, which can be given once a week, is under clinical trial. Byetta resembles GLP-1, a hormone produced by intestine, which is believed to promote the growth of new beta- cells in pancreas.
- **Insulin-sensitizer pills**, which are known as PPAR agonists (peroxisome proliferator activated receptor agonists) are being developed by a number of drug manufacturing companies.
- A new class of oral drugs called **DPP-IV** (dipeptidyl peptidase – iv) inhibitors, which boost the levels of glucose controlling hormones are also on clinical trials. These drugs also raise the levels of GLP-1.
- **Acomplia** blunts appetite by blocking brain receptors. This drug may prove very useful for the treatment of obesity.

Chapter 21

RECIPES FOR DIABETICS

Healthy diet is imperative for the management of diabetes. A diabetic patient need not feel that he is deprived of good food. Many books are available in present times, containing recipes designed especially for the diabetic patients. Many food exchanges as well as easy, quick and tasty meal preparations are available. Besides food preparations, the portion size, the calorie content and the nutritional value are critical elements in the day-to-day meal planning. Herein are details of some Indian recipes. These are different and unique in their flavors; have exotic taste, are addictive and intriguing. They contain fragrant herbs and rich blend of spices. Many different blends of spices are available in the Indian market.

Indian spices are also available in large supermarkets like the international Tops in USA. In USA, spices are also available in Indian stores. Many of these spices have medicinal value too and some of the preparations given here are recommended in Ayurvedic texts for diabetics. Besides, being low in calorie content, they are rich in fibers and are nutritional. They are quick and easy to make with readily available ingredients. **Curry**, a commonly used word, simply means gravy.

The authentic Indian cuisine gets its distinctive subtle or strident taste by virtue of spices. Ginger and garlic are added frequently to the preparations. Turmeric is also a very commonly used ingredient. In fact, all curries have a rich blend of turmeric. Ghee, which is derived from butter, is used in traditional Indian cooking. However, it is advisable to use olive oil or canola oil. Refined mustard oil, which is also available in the market is also good and can be used in certain dishes.

It is better to use non-stick cooking pans as these significantly lower the quantity of fat used. Lentils or dals as called in Hindi, form a part of staple diet in India. Urad dal, also known as black gram bean, is used as whole or split i.e. without skin, quite frequently. Kala chana is related to chickpea, but different from it and has brown skin. Chana dal is split kala chana without skin. Among other lentils are toor dal, frequently used in south Indian preparations and mung dal also known as green gram. In the following preparations, the amount of spices can be reduced if a less hot preparation is preferred.

Lassi

This is a popular and a refreshing drink. It is taken anytime during the day with or without meal. It is a favorite, especially during summers. It is very easy to prepare and is healthy and very soothing.

Ingredients

1 cup nonfat yogurt (120 ml)
¼ teaspoon salt
¼ teaspoon black pepper
artificial sweetener to taste and crushed ice.

Whisk all the ingredients in a blender until frothy and serve over ice.

Serving 2 = Calorie per serving 60,
Protein 6 gm,
Fat 0 gm,
Carbohydrate 9 gm.

Nimbu Adrak Pani

In Hindi, lime is called **nimbu**, ginger is called **adrak** and water is known as **pani**. This is a refreshing and invigorating drink, especially on a hot summer day.

Ingredients

Fresh limejuice of $^{2}/_{3}$ cup (80 ml)
1 tablespoon peeled
chopped fresh ginger
1 teaspoon black pepper
½ teaspoon salt
1 packet sweetener / 8 tablets of equal and crushed ice.

Put the ginger in a pan with a cup of water, boil it and simmer for few minutes. Strain the mixture into a pitcher, add salt, black pepper and sweetener and let it cool. Add limejuice and stir well. Chill the mixture. Before serving, add 4 cups of water and serve over crushed ice. The calorie content is negligible.

Adrak Elaichi Tea

Cardamom is called **illachi** in Hindi. This is an intoxicating beverage, more so in winter.

Ingredients

Water 4½ cups
½ teaspoon fresh grated ginger
2 green cardamom pods
milk/cream optional
sugar/sweetener optional 4 tea bags.

Put the water in a pan and bring it to boil. Then add ginger and ground cardamom seeds to the water, cover the pan with a lid and allow it to simmer over very low heat for 10-15 minutes. Sieve this into 4 cups, each containing one tea bag. Serve it hot. Milk/cream and sugar/ sweetener may be added, if desired.

Serving 4 = Calorie content is negligible if no milk
cream or sugar is added.

Raita

This is a cool, colorful and a healthy starter. It is quick and easy to prepare.

Ingredients

Plain nonfat yogurt 2 cups (240 ml)
1 small onion finely chopped
2 large tomatoes cut into cubes
1 fresh green chilli finely chopped (optional)
½ teaspoon salt, ½ teaspoon black pepper
1 tablespoon minced or finely chopped fresh mint leaves.

Place the yogurt in a bowl and whisk it until smooth. Add the remaining ingredients and stir lightly to combine. Cover and chill in the refrigerator until ready to serve. Addition of diced apple, pineapple, cucumber and/or cantaloupe can modify this preparation.

Serving 4 = Calorie per serving 80
Protein 8 gm
Fat 0 gm
Carbohydrate 12 gm

Sooji Uppma

Semolina or **sooji** as is called in Hindi, can be used to prepare a number of dishes. It is easy and quick to cook. It is a healthy ingredient and can be served in a variety of ways as a snack or regular meal. Uppma is a popular and a tasty dish.

Ingredients

1 tablespoon cooking oil
1 tablespoon split urad dal 1 tablespoon split chana dal
½ teaspoon salt or to taste
½ teaspoon cumin seeds
½ teaspoon red pepper powder (optional)
½ teaspoon mustard seeds
1 black cardamom
4 cloves
1 small onion finely chopped
1 cup frozen mixed vegetables or green peas
1 cup semolina
4 fresh curry leaves Fresh chopped coriander leaves to garnish.

Heat half the oil in non-stick pan over moderate heat and add semolina. Stir gently till the semolina is light brown and there is a fragrant smell. Put it aside. Heat the remaining oil in a separate pan and add mustard seeds and stir-fry until they crackle. Add both **dals** and stir until they are golden brown. Add the remaining spices and fry for few minutes. Add vegetables and 3 cups of water and bring it to boil. Add semolina and cook over moderate heat till water is totally absorbed. Garnish with coriander.

Servings 6 = Calories per serving-200
Protein 6 gm
Fat 4gm
Carbohydrate 35 gm

Palak Paneer

Spinach called **palak** in Hindi is a rich source of iron and fiber. *Paneer* is cottage cheese compressed into a cake. It is a rich source of protein with very little fat in it. In India, this dish forms part of a major meal that generally includes yogurt, *dal* and **chappatis** (bread resembling tortilla). In case paneer is not available, it can be substituted by equal amount of ricotta cheese.

Ingredients

2 packages (8oz each) frozen chopped spinach
2 packages (8oz each)
low fat cheese or cake of cottage cheese cut into cubes
1 tablespoon cooking oil or mustard oil
1-teaspoon cumin seeds
½ teaspoon mustard seeds
½ teaspoon red pepper
½ teaspoon salt
½ teaspoon minced garlic.

Heat the oil in non-stick pan over moderate heat. Add mustard seeds and fry until they crackle. Add cumin seeds, salt, pepper and garlic and fry for about 2 minutes or till garlic is light brown. Add spinach and cheese and cook till water dries up. A packet of dried kastoori methi (fenugreek) about 50 gm can be substituted for garlic. Garlic is a good anti-oxidant whereas fenugreek is anti-diabetic.

Serving 6 = Calorie per serving 80
Protein 8 gm
Fat 3gm
Carbohydrate 5 gm

Ginger Garlic Halibut

Fish is one of the best form of proteins. Both ginger and garlic are anti-oxidants. It is a healthy and tangy preparation.

Ingredients

Halibut steaks 4
1 teaspoon garlic paste
1 teaspoon ginger paste
¼ teaspoon salt
1 teaspoon black pepper.

In a small bowl, combine both the pastes with salt and pepper. Give fine knife cuts in the fish and smear the paste into the cuts and all over the fish. Spray a baking sheet with nonstick cooking spray. Wrap in the steaks in the baking sheet, putting the steaks side by side. Preheat the oven to 350° F. Bake the fish for 10-15 minutes. This method of cooking allows the essential flavors of the fish to be preserved. Serve it hot with lemon slices.

Serving 4 = Calorie per serving 130
Protein 24 gm
Fat 3 gm
Carbohydrate 2 gm.

Spinach Salmon

Salmon is a rich source of omega-3 fatty acids. Spinach besides having fiber has high iron content. Fenugreek used in the dish is good for diabetes.

Ingredients

4 salmon fillets
1 package of spinach (8oz) thawed
1 package of fenugreek (8oz) thawed
¼ teaspoon mustard seeds
¼ teaspoon fenugreek seeds
1 tablespoon mustard oil
¼ teaspoon salt

1 teaspoon black pepper
1 tablespoon vinegar.

Put the oil in a nonstick pan and heat over moderate heat. Add mustard seeds and heat until the seeds crackle. Add salt, pepper, fenugreek seeds and stir-fry till fenugreek seeds turn golden brown or just a shade darker. Add spinach and fenugreek leaves, mix the two and cook for few minutes. Spread salmon fillets on the leaves. Add vinegar. Cover the pan and cook for 15-20 minutes or till the water dries up and the fish flakes.

Serving 4 = Calories per serving 280
Proteins 30 gm
Fat 15 gm
Carbohydrate 4 gm

Ginger Lime Salmon

Ingredients

4 salmon steaks
2 tablespoon fresh limejuice
¼ teaspoon salt
1 teaspoon ginger paste
1 tablespoon butter

Preheat the broiler. Coat the broiler pan with nonstick cooking spray. Place the salmon in the pan. In a small bowl, mix the remaining ingredients. Spread the mixture evenly over the salmon steaks. Broil for 10-15 minutes.

Serving 4 = Calories per serving 360
Proteins 36 gm
Fat 22 gm
Carbohydrate 4 gm.

Tandoori Chicken

This is a famous north Indian preparation, loved and relished by all. It has distinctive orange-red color and cooked in a traditional Indian tandoor, an oven like devise. The present recipe is modified and prepared in conventional oven.

Ingredients

Four whole boneless chicken breasts without the skin
½ cup fresh lemon juice
½ cup plain nonfat yogurt
½ teaspoon salt
1 teaspoon red pepper
1 teaspoon cumin powder
1 teaspoon coriander powder
½ teaspoon cardamom powder
½ teaspoon turmeric powder
1 tablespoon garlic paste
2 tablespoon paprika
1 tablespoon ginger paste
Cooking oil spray.

With a sharp knife, make slashes in the chicken breasts, about ½ inch deep and 1 inch apart. Rub salt and lemon juice into the cuts and put the chicken aside in a shallow dish. Put the remaining ingredients in blender and blend them coarsely without over processing. Rub this marinade into the chicken thoroughly. Place it in the refrigerator and allow it to marinade overnight. Preheat the oven to 450° F. Place the chicken on a wire rack in a large roasting pan. Spray oil on the chicken and cook it in the oven for 20-25 minutes or until it is tender.

Serving 4 = Calorie per serving 300
Protein 62 gm
Fat 4 gm
Carbohydrate 2gm.

Roasted Chicken

This is a quick, simple and delicious recipe. It is somewhat similar to the previous preparation, but it is less spicy.

Ingredients

Four boneless chicken breasts without skin
½ cup fresh lemon juice
½ cup nonfat plain yogurt
½ teaspoon salt
½ teaspoon red pepper
2 tablespoon tomato puree.

Make slashes with a sharp knife into the chicken as in the previous recipe. Mix all the remaining ingredients except the tomato puree and rub the mixture over and into the chicken pieces in a bowl. Put it into the refrigerator and leave it to marinade for 2 hours. After marinating, smear the tomato puree on the chicken breasts and transfer them into a roasting pan. Roast it in a preheated oven at 450° F for 20-25 minutes or until the chicken is tender.

Serving 4 = Calorie content and nutritional values are the same as in the previous recipe.

Bitter Gourd

In Ayurvedic text, preparations of bitter gourd are considered very good for diabetics. The juice extracted from fresh gourd is very effective but also very bitter and patients tend to discontinue with it because of the taste. Cooked preparations are more palatable. There are several methods of preparing this vegetable. The method described here can be modified to suit individual tastes.

Ingredients

Bitter gourd ½ pound
1 medium onion coarsely sliced
1 tablespoon tomato puree
½ teaspoon cumin seeds
a packet of sweetener
½ teaspoon dried mango powder (amchor)
1 teaspoon salt
2 tablespoon cooking oil.

Clean, peel and seed the gourd by making a vertical slit. Smear each piece with salt and keep them in a plate, overnight in the refrigerator. Wash and pat dry the gourd. Cut them transversely into ½ inch long pieces. Heat the oil in a nonstick saucepan over moderate heat. Add cumin and stir-fry for few minutes. Add gourd and continue to stir-fry until the pieces turn light brown. Add onion and stir-fry until onion becomes golden brown. Add tomato puree, sugar and dried mango powder. Stuffing the long pieces of gourd with mashed potatoes, instead of cutting them transversely, can modify the dish.

Serving 4 = Calorie per serving 80
Protein 3 gm
Fat 4 gm
Carbohydrate 8 gm

Onion Okra

It is a delicious and spicy dish. The secret of a good preparation is to use fresh and not frozen okra. It is a part of the main meal and taken with Indian bread or chappati.

Ingredients

Fresh okra 8 oz
2 tablespoon cooking oil
1 large onion
2 green chilies
½ teaspoon turmeric powder
½ teaspoon salt
½ teaspoon garam masala
½ teaspoon paprika
2 garlic cloves crushed
1-inch fresh ginger grated.

With a sharp knife trim the tops of okra stems and cut each stem across into ½ inch bits. Cut the onion into long thin slices. Cut the chillies longitudinally into two halves each. Put the oil into thick base nonstick pan. Add garlic, ginger and fry for few minutes. Add onion and okra and cook over very low heat and stir gently. Add spices and chillies. Keep stirring and frying on low heat until the okra becomes soft and tender. Water is not added generally, so as to get a crispy preparation. However, if the okra starts sticking to the bottom of the pan, then sprinkle a little water. Serve it hot.

Serving 2 = Calories per serving 86
Protein 3 gm
Fat 4 gm
Carbohydrate 8 gm.

Urad Dal

Sabut urad dal or whole black gram is a nourishing and a very popular preparation of north India. Lot of butter is added to this dal when cooked in regular manner. However, in this recipe butter has been totally omitted to cut down the calories and fat. Towards the end of the preparation, a cup of milk is added to give it a rich taste. Some prefer to add ½ cup of yogurt instead of milk. Addition of green chilies and generous use of ginger gives it a distinctive taste.

Ingredients

1 cup whole black gram
1 tablespoon red kidney beans
1 tablespoon fresh grated ginger
½ teaspoon minced garlic
½ onion finely chopped
2 tablespoon cooking oil
salt to taste
½ teaspoon red pepper
½ teaspoon garam masala
2 fresh green chillies finely chopped.

Soak beans and black gram in a bowl filled with water to a level 2 inch above the dal level and leave it overnight. Next morning, drain the water, if any. Next, put the dal and beans with salt in a saucepan. Add three cups of water and cook till the dal is soft and mushy. This can also be done in a pressure cooker. In a separate nonstick pan, heat the oil. Add onion to the oil and fry, while stirring, till onion becomes light brown and curls up. Add ginger and garlic and continue to fry, stirring all the time till the garlic becomes light brown. Add green chillies and few minutes later add red pepper. Then add the cooked dal mixture to the fried ingredients. Add garam masala. Add a cup of milk and continue to cook over low heat for few minutes. The final preparation should neither be too thick nor too watery.

Serving 4 = Calorie per serving 258
Protein 9 gm
Fat 6 gm
Carbohydrate 42 gm.

Red Kidney Beans

All types of beans are rich source of fibers, vitamin B and manganese. As detailed in previous section, manganese is an important trace mineral required for healthy bones and prevents osteoporosis. A diet rich in fibers is essential for proper gut motility, as the food tends to stagnate in the gut leading to excessive absorption of cholesterol into the blood, an important risk factor in heart disease. Dish of red kidney beans is healthy and nutritious. Eaten with plain boiled rice, it is fulfilling and quite a favorite in north India.

Ingredients

Two cups red kidney beans
1 teaspoon shredded fresh ginger
1 teaspoon minced garlic
1 onion finely chopped
2 tablespoon tomato puree
2 tablespoon cooking oil
2 fresh green chillies finely chopped
½ teaspoon red pepper
½ teaspoon garam masala
1 teaspoon salt

Place the beans in 3 cups of water and soak them overnight. Add 3 cups of water and salt to the beans and cook until the beans are soft and a little mushy. Do not overcook. This may be done in a pressure cooker or a saucepan. Keep the cooked beans aside. In a separate nonstick pan heat the oil over moderate heat. Add onion and stir-fry until onion is golden brown. Add garlic and ginger and continue to stir-fry until garlic turns a shade darker. Add tomato puree, red pepper and green chillies and cook for few minutes. Combine this mixture to the cooked beans and add garam masala. Serve it warm.

Serving 8 = Calorie per serving 230
Protein 10 gm
Fat 3 gm
Carbohydrate 40 gm.

Kaboli Chana

This is another tangy, spicy and addictive north Indian dish. It is popularly served with bhatura, a kind of deep fried puffed bread. When eaten with mango pickle and onion salad, it makes an intoxicating meal. Kaboli chana is like chickpeas.

Ingredients

Two cups whole dried chickpeas
2 tablespoon cooking oil
1 large onion finely chopped
1 tablespoon grated fresh ginger
1 teaspoon minced garlic
Salt to taste
½ teaspoon cumin seeds
1 teaspoon red pepper
1 tablespoon tomato puree
4 pods cardamom
1 teaspoon garam masala
1 tablespoon amchor (dried mango powder) and 1-packet tealeaves.

Put the chickpeas in a bowl and add 3 cups of water. Soak them overnight. Drain water if any. Put the chickpeas in a large saucepan and add 3 cups of water. Add salt and tealeaves packet and cook till chickpeas become soft but not overcooked. Keep it aside, removing the tea packet. In a separate nonstick pan, heat the oil on moderate heat. Put cumin seeds and stir-fry till they turn shade darker. Add onion and stir-fry till onion turns light brown. Add ginger and garlic and continue to fry. Add a teaspoon of water if the mixture tends to stick to the pan. Add red pepper and tomato puree. Now, combine the cooked chickpeas to the fried mixture and cook over moderate till the gravy is thick. At the end add garam masala, amchor and ground cardamom seeds.

Serving 6 = Calorie per serving 400
Protein 20 gm
Fat 12 gm3
Carbohydrate 52 gm.

Kala Chana

Kala chana resemble chickpeas but they are smaller and have dark brown skin. They constitute one of the healthiest foods.

Ingredients

Two cups *kala chana*
2 tablespoon cooking oil
1 small onion finely chopped
1 teaspoon ginger finely chopped
1 teaspoon-minced garlic
1 teaspoon cumin seeds
½ teaspoon red pepper
1 tablespoon tomato puree
½ teaspoon garam masala
salt to taste
pinch of asafetida.

Soak the **chana** overnight in 3 cups of water as in the previous recipe. Cook them in 3 cups of water, adding salt, until they are tender and there is small quantity of water left. In a separate nonstick pan heat the oil over moderate heat. Add cumin seeds and stir-fry till they become a shade darker. Add onion, garlic and ginger and continue to stir-fry until onion becomes light brown in color. Add tomato puree, red pepper, asafetida, and garam masala. Combine the cooked chana to the mixture in the pan and serve them hot.

Serving 6 = Calorie per serving 260
Proteins 10 gm
Fats 6 gm
Carbohydrate 40 gm.

Sambar

This is a favorite of both north and south Indians. It is a hot, spicy vegetable and lentil, stew like preparation. The basic ingredient in this recipe is toor dal. Served with rice, it forms a staple diet in south India. This preparation resembles sambhar, as it has been modified.

Ingredients

One cup split toor dal
1 tablespoon cooking oil
salt to taste
1 teaspoon turmeric powder
½ teaspoon red pepper
½ teaspoon cumin seeds
½ teaspoon fenugreek seeds
½ teaspoon black mustard seeds
¼ teaspoon ground asafetida
6 fresh curry leaves
6 dried red chillies
1 tablespoon sambar masala
1-inch ball of tamarind pulp
2 medium ripe tomatoes diced
1 medium eggplant cut into 1 inch cubes
½ pound okra trimmed and cut into 1inch cubes.

Put the lentil in nonstick saucepan and add 6 cups of water, salt and turmeric powder. Heat to boil and then reduce the heat and allow it to simmer till the dal is soft and broken. This can also be done in pressure cooker to save time. Set it aside.

Next, place the tamarind pulp in a bowl and soak it in a cup of hot water for about 20 minutes. Mash the pulp thoroughly with fingers, strain through a sieve and squeeze as much of the tamarind liquid as possible.

Heat the oil in a large nonstick saucepan over moderate heat. Add mustard seeds and stir-fry until they crackle. Add the fenugreek and cumin seeds, red chillies and curry leaves and stir for few minutes. Add sambar masala and asafetida. Add all the vegetables, tamarind liquid and red pepper powder. Let it simmer until the vegetables are tender.

Add dal and continue to stir. Simmer for about 5 minutes more. Serve it hot.

Serving 8 = Calorie per serving 140
Protein 7 gm
Fat 3 gm
Carbohydrate 20 gm.

Punjabi Kadhi

This is a delightful preparation, tangy and spicy, served with boiled rice and quite a favorite in north India. It is a yogurt based creamy sauce with chickpea flour dumplings floating in it. As chickpea dumplings are deep-fried and consume lot of oil, this recipe is modified from the traditional dish wherein the dumplings have been excluded and replaced by onion. Sour yogurt is used in this preparation. In case sour yogurt is not available, plain nonfat yogurt mixed with a pinch of yeast is left in a warm place for 6-8 hours or overnight for the yogurt to become sour. In place of yogurt, sour buttermilk can be used.

Ingredients

Two cups nonfat plain yogurt/buttermilk
2/3cup chickpea flour
1 teaspoon turmeric powder
1 teaspoon salt
1 teaspoon red pepper
½ teaspoon fenugreek seeds
½ teaspoon black mustard seeds
1 teaspoon cumin seeds
1 large onion coarsely cut longitudinally
2 fresh green chillies
sliced longitudinally
6 curry leaves
2 teaspoon cooking oil.

Place the yogurt in a food processor and run it for seconds. Add chickpea flour and 6 cups of water and run the machine to make a smooth mixture.

Take a large saucepan and heat the oil over moderate heat. Put mustard seeds in the oil and stir-fry till the seeds crackle. Add fenugreek and cumin seeds and stir-fry till their color darkens. Add turmeric powder, red pepper, salt, green chillies and onion. Sir-fry till onions get translucent. Combine the yogurt chickpea flour mixture to the fried mixture. Bring it to boil and lower the heat to minimum. Continue to stir to prevent curdling. Cook uncovered until the mixture is reduced to nearly half its original quantity. Add curry leaves towards the end of cooking to preserve their flavor. When the preparation is ready it is a smooth sauce. Serve it hot with rice.

Serving 6-8 = Calorie per serving 180
Protein 16 gm
Fat 4 gm
Carbohydrate 20 gm.

Sarson Ka Saag

This is a very favorite north Indian dish relished, especially in winter months and eaten with makka (corn) ki roti (tortilla like preparation). Sarson is mustard plant. It is cultivated in winter months in north India. It is harvested in the beginning of spring, its seeds are used to prepare mustard oil and leaves are consumed like spinach leaves. It is a healthy tasty dish rich in iron and fibers.

Ingredients

Sarson leaves 500 gm
Spinach leaves 250 gm
2-3 fresh green chillies
1 small onion
½ tsp. Red chilli powder
2cm piece ginger
2 tbsp oil
salt to taste
1 tbsp butter.

Wash spinach and sarson thoroughly and cut them into fine pieces. Cook in pressure cooker for ½ hour. Grind the sag and cook over low heat till it becomes a thick paste. Set it aside. Heat oil in saucepan, add finely copped green chillies, grated onion and grated ginger to the oil and stir fry till onion become light brown in color. Add sag paste, salt and red chilli powder to this and continue to cook on low heat for about 10 minutes. Garnish it with butter and serve it hot.

Serving 4-6: Calories per serving-120
Fat 4 gm
Carbohydrate 20 gm.

Sandesh

This is a soft textured, delicate Bengali sweet made from Indian cottage cheese. It can, similarly be prepared from ricotta cheese. It is served as desert or evening snack.

Ingredients

One pound ricotta or Indian cottage cheese
¼ cup sugar
20 thinly slivered pistachio nuts.

Put the cheese in a sieve and press to remove as much moisture as possible. In a blender, process the cheese until it smoothens. Place the cheese in a nonstick saucepan and heat it gently over low heat, stirring all the time until the cheese forms a solid mass. Remove from the heat and cool slightly. Add sugar and mix thoroughly with the cheese. Knead it and allow it to cool. When cool enough to handle, taking small portion of the mixture roll into 1-inch round balls. Place pistachio slivers on each ball and place the balls on wax paper. Store them in refrigerator and serve them cool. About 20 balls will form.

Calorie per ball 57
Protein 6 gm
Fat 1 gm
Carbohydrate 6 gm.

Sandesh

American [illegible]
www [illegible]
American [illegible]
American [illegible]
American [illegible]
Canada [illegible]
nlm [illegible]
Joslin [illegible]
Harvard [illegible]
Juvenile [illegible]
National [illegible]
(NIDDK) [illegible]
1995 [illegible]
diabetes [illegible]
National [illegible]
(NIDDK) [illegible]
Publication [illegible]
http [illegible]
National [illegible]
THE [illegible]
2diabetes [illegible]
University [illegible]
www [illegible]

American [illegible]
nephro [illegible]
Anderson [illegible]
supplement [illegible]
individuals [illegible]
Arch [illegible]

References

Internet Addresses

- American Association of Clinical Endocrinologists http://www.aace.com
- American Association of Diabetes Educators http://www.AADEnet.org
- American Diabetes Association http://www.diabetesnet.com/ada.html
- American Diabetic Association http://www.eatright.org
- Canadian Diabetes Association http://www.diabetes.ca/http://nlm.nih.gov/ftrs/default/browse?hitK=O&search
- Joslin Diabetes Center Home fructosamine test. http://wwwjoslin.Harvard.edu/education/library/ fructosamine-test.html.
- Juvenile Diabetes Foundation http://www.jdfcure.com
- National Institute of Diabetes and Digestive and Kidney Diseases (NIDDK). Diabetes Statistics. NIH Publication No. 96-3926. October 1995. Updated August 13, 1997. Available at http://www.niddk.nih.gov/dmstats/dmstats.html.
- National Institute of Diabetes and Digestive and Kidney Diseases (NIDDK). Diabetic Neuropathy: The Nerve Damage of Diabetes. NIH Publication No. 95-3185, July 1995, updated October 1999. Available at http://www.niddk.nih.gov/health/diabetes/pubs/neuro/neuro.html.
- National Institutes of Health http://www.niddk.nih.gov/
- THERPY OF DIABETES MALLITUS (Diet and exercise in type 2diabetes).
- University of Wisconsin Diabetes Knowledgebase http://www.biostat.wisc.edu. /diaknow.index.htm.

Papers Published on Journals

- American Diabetes Association Position Statement: Diabetes nephropathy. Diabetes Care 1998: 21 (Suppl 1): S50.
- Anderson RA, Cheng N, Bryden NA, et al. Elevated intakes of supplemental chromium improves glucose and insulin variables in individuals with type 2diabetes. Diabetes. 1997; 46: 1786-1791.
- Arch J. Korytkowski M. Strategies for preventing coronary heart disease

in diabetes mellitus. Diabetes Spectrum. 1999; 12: 88-94.

- Atkinson MA, Maclaren NK: The pathogenesis of insulin-dependant diabetes mellitus. N Eng J Med 1994; 331: 1428.
- Cheatham B, Kahn CR: Insulin action and the insulin-signaling network. Endo Rev 1995; 16: 117.
- Chen G, Koyama K, Yuan X, et al. Disappearance of body fat in normal rats induced by adenovirus-mediated leptin gene therapy. Proc. Natl. Acad. Sci. 1996; 93: 14795-14799.
- Colwell JA; The feasibility of intensive insulin management in non-insulin-dependent diabetes mellitus: Implications of the Veterans Affairs Cooperative Study on Glycemic Control and Complications in NIDDM.Ann Intern Med 1996; 124(1part2): 131.
- Cryer PE, Fisher JN, Shamoon H; Hypoglycemia. Diabetes Care'1994; 17:734.
- David Loshak; Elevated blood pressure among U.S. adults with diabetes 1994. Am J of Preventive Med 2002, 22(1) 42-44.
- Davidson MB, Peter AL; An overview of metformin in the treatment of type2diabetes mellitus. Am J Med 1997; 102:99
- Hattersley AT: Maturity onset diabetes of the young: Clinical heterogeneity explained by genetic heterogeneity. Diabetic Med 1998; 15: 15.
- Holleman F, HoekstraJB; Insulin Lispro. N Engl J Med 1997; 337:176.
- Johannsson G, Karlsson C, Lonn L, et al. Serum leptin concentration and insulin sensitivity in men with abdominal obesity. Obes. Res. 1998; 6: 416-421.
- Jovanovic-Peterson L.,Guitierrez M., Peterson C. Chromium supplementation for gestational diabetic women improves glucose tolerance and decreases hyperinsulinemia. Diabetes. 1996; 45 (suppl 2): 337A.
- Karam JH: Reversible insulin resistance in non-insulin-dependent Diabetes mellitus. Horm Metab Res 1996; 28:440
- Kelly DB, ed-in-chief. American Diabetes Association Complete Guide to Diabetes. Alexandria, VA: American Diabetes Association; 1996; 27-29. and 1996; 14.
- Lebovitz HE: Alpha-glucosidase inhibitors. Endocrinol Metab Clin North Am 1997; 26:5 Effect acrobose delay in digestion and absorption of complex carbohydrates
- Maggs DG et al: Metabolic effects of troglitazone monotherapy in type2diabetes Mellites. Ann Intern Med 1998: 128: 176.
- Maron D, Fazio S, Linton MF. Current perspectives on statins. Circulation. 2000; 101:207.

- Polonsky KS, Sturis J, Bell GI: Seminars in Medicine of the Beth Israel Hospital, Boston. Non-insulin-dependent diabetes mellitus-genetically programmed failure of beta cell to compansate for insulin resistance. N Engl J Medicine 1996; 334:777.
- Ravina A, Slezak L, Mirsky N, Bryden NA, Anderson RA. Reversal of corticosteroid-induced diabetes mellitus with supplemental chromium. Diabetic Medicine. 1999; 16: 164-167.
- Ryan EA. Pancreas transplant for whom? [commentary]. Lancet. 1998; 351: 1072-1073.
- Scandinavian Simvastatin Survival Study Group. Randomized trial of cholesterol lowering in 4444 patients with coronary heart disease: the Scandinavian Simvastatin Survival Study (45). Lancet. 1994; 344: 1383-1389.
- Shapiro AMJ, Lakey JRT, Ryan EA, et al. Islet transplantation in seven patients with type 1diabetes mellitus using a glucocorticoid-free immunosuppressive regimen. N Engl J Med. 2000; 343: 230-238.
- United Kingdom Prospective Diabetes Study 24: Ann Intern Med 1998: 128: 165.
- Yamashita S ET al: Insulin resistance and body fat distribution: Contribution of visceral fat accumulation to development of insulin resistance and arteriosclerosis. Diabetic care 1996; 19:287.

Various Research Groups

- American Diabetes Association. Clinical Practice Recommendation 2000. Gestational diabetes mellitus. Diabetes Care. 2000; 23 (Suppl 1): S77-S79.
- American Diabetes Association. Clinical Practice Recommendation 2000. Diabetic retinopathy. Diabetes Care. 2000; 23 (Suppl 1): S73-S76
- American Diabetic Association. Clinical Practice Recommendation 2000. Management of dyslipidemia in adults with diabetes. Diabetes Care. 2000, 23(suppl 1): S57-S60.
- American Diabetic Association: Clinical Practice recommendations 1998. Diabetic Care 1998; 21(Suppl): S1
- American Diabetic Association: Nutrition recommendations and principles for the patients with diabetes mellitus (Position statement.) Diabetes Care 1998; 21(Suppl): S32 (Major changes in nutritional therapy of diabetes include the elimination of "ADA diet prescriptions," allowing freer substitution of sucrose in the meals and recommending tailored prescriptions for each diabetic patient based on individual goals.)
- DCCT Research Group: Hypoglycemia in the Diabetes Control and Complications Trial Diabetes 1997; 46:271.

- DCCT Research Group: The effect of intensive treatment of diabetes on the development and progression of long-term complications in insulin-dependent diabetes mellitus. New Engl J Med. 1993; 329: 977-986.
- DCCT Research Group: The relationship of glycemic exposure (HbA1c) to the risk of development and progression of retinopathy in the DCCT. Diabetes: 1995;44: 968-983.

Reference Books

- 101 Tips for Staying Healthy with Diabetes, by the University of New Mexico Diabetes Care Group. (1996)
- Anatomy by Ernest W. April. National Medical Series from Williams & Wilkins. Baltimore.
- Diabetes A to Z, by the American Diabetes Association (Rev. 1996)
- Diabetes for Dummies by Alan L. Rubin, M.D. I.D.G. books Worldwide Inc. An International data book company.
- Dieting for Dummies by Jane Kirby,R.D., I.D.G. books Worldwide Inc. An International data book company.
- Harper's Biochemistry by R.K. Murray, D.K. Granner, P.A. Mayes and V.W. Rodwell. Appleton and Lange, Norwalk, Connecticut/ San Mateo, California.
- Last's text book of Anatomy,edited by R.M.H. McMinn, M.D., PhD, FRCS., English Language Book Society/ Churchill Livingstone.
- Light on Yoga. By BKS Iyengar., London Unwin Paperbacks.
- Managing Diabetes on a Budget, by Leslie Y. Dawson. ADA. (1995)
- Natural Alternatives to Over-the-Counter and Prescription Drugs, by Michael T. Murray, N.D. William Morrow and Company inc. N.Y.
- Physiology by John Bullock, Joseph Boyle, 111, and Michael B. Wang. National Medical Series from Williams & Wilkins. Baltimore.
- Practical Guide to Diabetes Management by William T. Cefalu, M.D., Medical Information Press, New York.
- Reversing Diabetes, by Julian Whitaker, M.D. (1987)
- Textbook of Physiology and Biochemistry by George H Bell, J Norman Davidson and Harold Scarborough. The English Language Book Society and E. & S. Livingstone.
- The Diabetic's Book, by June Biermann and Barbara Toohey.
- The Johns Hopkins Guide to Diabetes, by Christopher D. Saudek, M.D., Richard R. Rubin, Ph.D. and Cynthia S. Shump, R.D., C.D.E. (1997)
- Yoga-101 essential tips, by Sivananda Yoga Vedanta Centre. Dorling Kindersley. N.Y.